Additional books by Catherine M. Poole

Melanoma: Prevention, Detection and Treatment, Catherine Poole with DuPont Guerry IV, MD. New Haven, CT: Yale University Press, 1998 and revised edition, 2005.

Choosing a Nurse-Midwife, Catherine M. Poole and Elizabeth A. Parr, CNM. New York: John Wiley and Sons, 1994.

Melanoma–
Not Just Skin Cancer

Catherine M. Poole

ISBN: 1502446553
ISBN 13: 9781502446558

Library of Congress Control Number: 2014917059
CreateSpace Independent Publishing Platform
North Charleston, South Carolina

To Patricia Garcia-Prieto—our time together was way too short! We were instant kindred spirits and sisters. We understood the needs of melanoma patients and how much work there was to do! She urged me to write this book and so here it is, another tool for melanoma patients. Patricia will remain foremost in my heart and soul as I continue this important work of helping melanoma patients.

Acknowledgments

I couldn't have written this update without the uncon-
ditional love and support from my husband, Stuart,
my horse Curley, and our farm family. My children, Jesse and
Carey, and grandchild, Declan, are always an inspiration to
me. The people who really spurred me on to update my previous work are the countless melanoma patients and caregivers I have worked with throughout the years at Melanoma
International Foundation (MIF). I know how frightening
and confusing the information about melanoma can be and
hope this book empowers patients to seek the best treatment.
I greatly appreciate those who shared their personal stories
to help others, both here and in the MIF video. In addition,
I am grateful to the MIF staff, Lisa, Alison, Jessi, volunteers,
advisory board, and scientific advisory board for continu-
ously working hard to maintain this foundation's excellent
reputation.

Let me also take this opportunity to express my gratitude
to all the extremely busy people who took the time to help me
with this book: Keith Flaherty, MD, and Jedd Wolchok, MD,

are brilliant, caring pioneers on the melanoma front who contributed their expertise on the newest therapies. DuPont Guerry, MD will always influence my thinking and writing about melanoma, but I'm happy he's taken a sabbatical from this one and is enjoying his well-deserved retirement. The support of my best friend Deborah, keeps me grounded.

Melanoma-
Not Just Skin Cancer

Catherine M. Poole

Contributors: Keith Flaherty, MD;
DuPont Guerry, MD; and Jedd Wolchok, MD

Contents

Acknowledgments vii

Foreword. xiii

Preface xv

1   What Is Melanoma?. 1

2   Who Gets Melanoma and Why? 9

3   Finding Early Melanoma. 27

4   If You Have Melanoma 41

5   When Melanoma Metastasizes 67

6   The Patient Experience: The Stories 97

7   Tending to Your Spirits. 115

Glossary 129

About the Author. 137

Notes. 139

Index. 143

Foreword

*I*n our collaboration on previous books on melanoma, I have described Catherine Poole as a practical, no-nonsense person and praised her for writing a practical, no-nonsense guide for patients—and their families and friends—dealing with melanoma. She has done it again, this time focusing on the ongoing translation of two kinds of elegant scientific discoveries into breakthrough therapies. The first of these was the uncovering of at least some of the molecular mistakes in the wiring of melanoma cells, and the second was the beginning of the clarification of the complex and shifting relationship of the immune system with such malignant cells as they grow and shape-shift. New technologies, new styles of collaboration between laboratory and clinical scientists in academia and in pharmaceutical companies, more efficient clinical trials, and the enfranchisement of energized patients have led to new drugs to deal with the miswiring problem (targeted therapy) and with melanoma cells that hide from the immune system, blind it, or suppress it (immunotherapy).

In this book, Catherine describes the right path—or paths—from the wise perspective of someone who has had melanoma and has enlisted the help of some of the physician-investigators leading the discovery and testing of new therapies. In addition, she is an experienced patient navigator for the Melanoma International Foundation, the wonderful organization she started. This personal and professional experience lends her book clarity, authenticity, spirit, and utility.

Much good has already come from these collaborations, scientific discoveries, and new drugs. But much still needs to be done to get us to where we need to go—to make melanoma a disease for which prevention is a mainstay, a cure is common, and long-term suppression is the worst outcome that can be expected. We have already learned enough to know that we are on the right path.

—DuPont Guerry IV, MD

Preface

I write this update to my melanoma book during a very busy time in my life. Running a foundation is very similar to running a business—you wear many hats! Having a grandson is great fun, too, and I didn't want to miss out on that. But I knew some patients and caregivers needed information that went beyond the Internet, so I decided to find the extra time for this book. There is still so much going on in clinical trials and in combinations of approaches that could be the home run we need. I am very thankful for the renewed interest in melanoma research! Most of all, I hope this book will turn panic into peaceful pursuance of the best possible therapy for melanoma patients. Having an electronic version will allow me to make future updates, and I'm excited that we may have more answers soon. I have to agree with Dr. Guerry when he states in the Foreword that we are on the right path. By utilizing this book as your companion, as well as the navigation services of the Melanoma International Foundation, you no longer need to travel that path alone.

CHAPTER 1

What Is Melanoma?

*I*n the early 1900s, the United States experienced a sweeping tide of radical social change. Society loosened up, and fashion followed the shift in attitude: more skin was bared. Hats and gloves, which had been a mainstay of fashion, were now discarded. Meanwhile, men took to wearing shorter collars and sleeves, and some shaved their beards and mustaches, eventually finding it acceptable to go shirtless in the summer sun. Within a few decades, pallor was no longer fashionable and suntans came into vogue, associated with higher social status. People coated their skin in baby oil and applied suntan lotion to get the "darkest, deepest tan." Sunlamps became a home beauty accessory. Tanning salons became the hot spot for teens to go before the prom. The historical trend toward increased sun and tanning lamp exposure, driven by the desire to darken one's skin, may help explain, in large part, the upswing in melanoma rates.

Skin: Your Body's Largest Organ

To understand what melanoma is and how it develops, it is helpful to understand basic anatomy and the function of the skin. Generally, skin isn't considered a functioning organ like the liver or the brain. Actually, most people don't realize that their skin is an organ at all. They understand that their skin protects them from excessive heat, cold, and other stimuli, but not that they need to protect it. The skin is, however, the largest organ of the body—responsible for shielding the rest of the body from excessive light and extreme temperatures, and guarding the body from infection and injury.

The skin's secondary role is social. It is one of the major ways we present ourselves to others. We work hard to adorn or improve our skin by applying makeup to it, having it pierced, or undergoing cosmetically corrective plastic surgery. Yet human skin can't compare with the hides of the rest of the animal kingdom. According to Dr. Wallace Clark, "Even were you to be arrayed with less spectacular creatures such as the… spotted skunk, the unadorned skin of Homo sapiens are by comparison, a scenic disaster."[1]

Any animal's epidermis not only serves an aesthetic function but also provides an extra layer of protection from the sun. Again, according to Dr. Clark, our skin structure is closest to that of pigs: "Only swine have the same organization of the dermis (inner layer of skin) as humans. Also like humans, swine enjoy lying in the sun, tan in response to the sun, and will drink beer in large quantities."[2]

Human skin is made up of two layers: the *dermis*, or inner layer, and the *epidermis*, or outer layer. Below the dermis is the fatty, or subcutaneous, layer (the *subcutis*). The dermis is divided into an upper part, called the *papillary dermis*, and a lower part, called the *reticular dermis*. The dermis contains several different types of cells and fibrous tissues along with blood and lymph vessels that nourish the epidermis, the outer layer where most skin cancers evolve. In the lower region of the epidermis are the *melanocytes*, which are cells that make a dark pigment called melanin that contributes to skin coloring. The melanocytes feed the melanin pigment to cells in the upper layer of skin, called *keratinocytes*. This provides them and the underlying structures with a natural sunblock of sorts.

Melanoma is the uncontrolled growth of melanocytes in one spot, thought to be set off by some of the ultraviolet wavelengths in sunlight (and sometimes other influences). If left to its natural course, a single melanoma can eventually penetrate from the epidermis into the dermis and adapt to growing there. Once melanoma spreads to the dermis, it has access to blood and lymph vessels—the freeways to the rest of the body. Therefore, if the melanoma reaches the dermis and is able to flourish, its cells have the potential to spread to other areas of the body. The dermis is where melanoma takes on its role as a full-fledged malignancy.

Types of Melanoma

Melanoma is a form of skin cancer, not to be confused with the more common squamous cell or basal cell skin cancers. These very common skin cancers arise from keratinocytes in the epidermis and are also triggered by sun exposure, yet they seldom become life threatening. In contrast, melanoma has a much higher potential to spread to other parts of the body and become a life-threatening illness.

There are several different types of melanoma, and *superficial spreading melanoma* is the most common, making up 70 to 80 percent of all cases. Although it is most frequently found on women's legs and on men's and women's backs, it can arise anywhere on the body, including areas never exposed to the sun. This type of melanoma often develops from an existing mole, but it can also come from an unblemished bit of skin. It is a brown-black spreading stain, usually at least half a centimeter (about a quarter of an inch) in diameter.

Nodular melanoma accounts for 10 percent of all melanoma cases. It occurs in the same locations on the body as superficial spreading melanoma, also frequently arises from a mole, and is a bit more common in men than in women. This type of melanoma is raised and dome shaped, sometimes resembling a blood blister. Both nodular and superficial spreading melanomas appear to be triggered by the combination of excessive intermittent sun exposure and skin sensitivity, which can be seen in the tendency toward sunburns.

Lentigo maligna melanoma is less common than either of the other two types, and is usually seen in older people. It is most commonly found on the face and other parts of the body that are chronically exposed to the sun. It develops after many years of heavy sun exposure and first appears as a dark and irregularly shaped stain. This type of melanoma does not develop from moles.

Acral lentiginous melanoma appears most frequently on the palms of the hands or the soles of the feet, on the under-surface of the fingers or toes, and under the nails. When it affects the nails, the melanoma begins at the base and makes a streak that extends to the tip of the nail. The thumbs and big toes are most often affected. It is not attributed to sun exposure. Most of the melanomas already mentioned appear predominantly in white people and are attributed to sun exposure, whereas acral lentiginous melanoma occurs in approximately the same frequency among whites and people of color; both at a low rate with an unknown causal factor. This is the type of melanoma that killed reggae music star Bob Marley in 1981. According to the *Philadelphia Inquirer,* Marley had acral lentiginous melanoma of his big toe, which spread to his lungs and brain.[3]

Mucosal melanoma appears on the mucous membranes of the body—inside the mouth and in the anal-genital region. It is a rare form of melanoma whose cause is unknown but that, given its location, is also assumed to be unrelated to sun exposure.

Another uncommon melanoma, *ocular melanoma,* arises at the back of the eye. Its cause, too, is unclear, since this area is well protected from the harmful wavelengths of sunlight by the cornea and lens. Even so, medical investigators speculate that ultraviolet radiation, especially in childhood, may pass through the front of the eye and trigger this rare kind of melanoma later in life. It commonly appears as a small freckle beneath the retina, and can grow and eventually spread to other organs of the body. As with all cancer, it is best to find ocular melanoma early and the best way is by periodic dilated retinal examination by an ophthalmologist. Ocular melanoma is definitely best treated by an eye specialist who deals with this disease regularly.

Occurring in an exception of cases, melanomas of all kinds can present themselves as *amelanotic* (without melanin pigment). These melanomas are difficult to recognize because they don't have the characteristic darkness of melanoma, but rather show up as clear, pink, or red growths. So if you have a new lesion, or one that grows and changes yet lacks that characteristic blackness of melanoma, it is still important to get it checked!

When Melanoma Becomes Malignant

A melanoma lesion isn't born malignant; in other words, it doesn't possess the ability to spread to the internal organs until it has progressed through certain growth phases. Dr. Clark coined the term *radial growth phase.* In this phase, the melanoma is *nontumorigenic*—that is, it doesn't form a tumor or lump or nodule. This phase actually comprises two steps: In the first, the melanoma cells are contained entirely in the epidermis. The cancer is thus described by the Latin term *in situ*, meaning "in place." In the second step, the invasive radial growth phase, the melanoma cells may invade the dermis on a very small scale, but do not flourish there, so the cancer is no longer regarded as being in situ. During this phase, the melanoma apparently can't send out cells to other parts of the body; still, if not recognized and removed, it will commonly proceed to the next step.

The next step or progression of a lesion's growth is called the *vertical growth*, or *tumorigenic*, phase. At this point, the melanoma begins to grow as a tumor in the dermis, in the form of an expanding sphere made up of abnormal melanocytes. During this step, there is some chance that the cancer may spread beyond the skin to other parts of the body. To prevent it from becoming life threatening, it is essential to obliterate the growth while it is in its flat (radial growth) phase before it gets to the lumpy (vertical growth) phase.[4]

To catch melanoma in its early phases, it is important to know the "look" of the lesion and understand the importance of any changes in it. The changes to look for make up the ABCDs of melanoma: **A**symmetry, **B**order irregularity, **C**olor variation, and a **D**iameter greater than six millimeters. Because with some early melanomas the skin is also slightly elevated or thickened, we can also add an E for **E**levation. If you're familiar with what is and isn't the normal "look" of your skin and that of your loved ones, you will be better armed to recognize melanoma at an early, curable stage. You just need to look for any change.

CHAPTER 2

Who Gets Melanoma and Why?

*E*pidemiologists have pinpointed certain characteristics that, whether they occur separately or in conjunction, predict who is likely to get melanoma. The predisposing factors include

- a sun-sensitive skin type that may freckle easily
- a history of spending too much time in the sun
- having lots of common moles or any "funny-looking" (dysplastic) moles
- a personal or family history of any of the common kinds of skin cancer (squamous and basal cell carcinoma)
- a personal or family history of melanoma

Other less important yet influential factors are gender, geographical location, and age. The risk of developing melanoma associated with each factor is in itself not great; however, for those individuals who possess multiple predisposing factors, the risk may be dramatically increased.

The Role of the Sun and Ultraviolet Radiation

The sun emits three types of electromagnetic radiation that are of concern to us: visible, infrared, and ultraviolet (UV). *Visible radiation* is the light we see; *infrared radiation* gives off warmth; and *UV radiation* is an invisible type that seems to have the greatest potential for deleterious biological effects. UV radiation is divided into three wavelengths: UV-A, UV-B, and UV-C. Only UV-A and UV-B reach the Earth's surface and can therefore directly assault your skin. UV radiation is a carcinogen, capable of both initiating a malignancy and promoting its growth and evolution. Although UV-B is thought to be the major carcinogenic agent in the formation of melanoma as well as nonmelanoma cancers, UV-A also makes a contribution. Light in both wave bands produces sunburns, along with the resultant skin damage, and accelerates the skin changes associated with aging, such as wrinkling and loss of elasticity.

Melanin pigment in the skin serves a protective role by absorbing and detoxifying UV radiation. The sensitivity of different skin types to sunburn and other photodamaging effects is genetically determined and significantly related to how melanin is packaged and distributed in skin cells—factors that also largely determine skin type and color.

Which Skin Types Are Susceptible to Melanoma?

Melanoma almost exclusively affects people with white skin; the only important exceptions, as mentioned in chapter 1, are acral lentiginous melanoma and mucosal melanoma, which affect people of all skin colors and bear no relation to sun exposure as far as we know. Freckles are an important barometer of both sun sensitivity and sun damage. A person who freckles easily has about twice the risk of getting melanoma as someone with no scattering of the telltale dots.

Some people have skin so sensitive that it turns a flaming shade of red when exposed to the sun for even a brief time. Usually their hair is red or blond, and their skin is porcelain white. (It is possible, though, to have dark hair and very fair skin.) Such skin, known as type 1, is the most likely to develop melanoma. There are four skin types: type 1, very pale; type 2, light white; type 3, olive to light brown; and type 4, brown to dark brown. These types are determined by tanning ability.

What Types of Sun Exposure Cause Melanoma?

UV radiation from sunlight not only burns the skin but also affects the DNA, or genetic material, in skin cells. Current wisdom holds that both kinds of UV, A and B, foster melanoma development, but it is UV-B that does the critical damage to certain genes in melanocytes that makes melanoma start. UV radiation may also have other far-reaching consequences, such as suppression of some functions of the immune system that retard tumor formation.

The most common kinds of melanoma, superficial spreading and nodular, seem to be associated with heavy, intermittent exposure to the sun, occurring in such situations as a person spending most of his time indoors but getting big doses of sun on vacations and weekends. Also, the *BRAF* gene mutation of tumors found in 50% of patients is linked to heavy sun exposure. One of the best definitions of BRAF can be found inThe Genetics Home Reference of the U.S. National Library of Medicine (http://ghr.nlm.nih.gov/gene/BRAF) which states "the *BRAF* gene belongs to a class of genes known as oncogenes. When mutated, oncogenes have the potential to cause normal cells to become cancerous." The discovery of this mutation has led to new BRAF inhibitor therapeutic options discussed later in the book Intermittent sun exposure at any time in a person's life, but particularly in childhood, increases the risk of skin cancer and the two most common kinds of melanoma. Study results conflict about whether sun exposure in childhood is associated with later melanoma because of a special vulnerability of the young or because children simply spend more time out in the sun. It is important to realize that no matter your age, getting too much sun can cause skin cancer.[1]

Intermittent intense exposure of untanned skin to sunlight is an important risk factor, but it is not the only kind of sun exposure that poses a threat. Lentigo maligna melanoma is associated with long-term exposure to the sun. This kind of melanoma often afflicts older people—especially men—who have heavily sun-damaged skin. It commonly occurs on the face and ears.

What about Tanning Salons?

According to the tanning industry websites, 28 million Americans patronize tanning salons, including 2.3 million teens. Most dermatologists strongly advise against relying on artificial sunlight to get a tan. The light tubes in tanning beds produce UV-A, the wavelength implicated in prematurely aging skin and in causing nonmelanoma skin cancers. This kind of light may also collude with UV-B to trigger melanoma. Also, a UV-A tan does not protect against UV-B damage. That is, a "base tan" obtained at a tanning salon won't protect you from burning when you go outdoors.. And although the tanning industry claims its facilities can provide vitamin D, which many people lack, experts maintain that taking vitamin D supplements and spending twenty minutes daily in the "real" sun will replenish this vitamin in those who are at risk of becoming deficient.

In 1994, the American Medical Association advocated the banning of artificial tanning, and in 2009, the World Health Organization moved UV tanning beds into its highest cancer-risk category. Brazil was the first country to ban tanning salons in 2009. However, the tanning industry—which now has profits of $5 billion per year—has learned to become an effective lobbyist against regulations of its industry. Since enforcement is still an issue once tanning laws are passed, regulations aren't the key to making tanning facilities safer. A start to doing so is the recent age restriction banning people under eighteen from receiving artificial tans, which has helped raise parents' awareness that this is not a safe activity. Banning salons altogether would be 100 percent more effective, as it might save millions of lives.

Are Bottled or Spray-on Tans Safe?

Some people maintain that bottled, or spray-on, chemically colored tans are the only safe tans. Commercial tanning formulas work by dying the top layers of skin, affecting only dead skin cells. Sunless tanning coats your skin with the chemical dihydroxyacetone (DHA), which interacts with the dead surface cells in the epidermis to darken skin color and simulate a tan. DHA should not be inhaled, ingested, or applied to areas covered by mucous membranes, including the lips, nose, and areas in and around the eye (from the top of the cheek to above the eyebrow) because the risks, if any, are unknown. Most sunless tanning sprays and lotions do not contain a skin-protecting sunscreen.

Is All Sun Exposure Bad?

Mild exposure to the sun is beneficial for most people. Indeed, it may have healthy effects: it helps to activate vitamin D, and can also lift one's spirits. It has been reported that the sort of mild, continual sun exposure that produces a bit of a tan but no burn may even protect you from melanoma. This modest protection comes at some cost, however. Sun exposure at minimal levels ages the skin and can precipitate non-melanoma skin cancers, of which there are estimated to be more than one million new cases per year.

What Are Moles?

In the medical world, moles are referred to as *nevi* (singular *nevus*). The average white adult may count about twenty-five moles, with the heaviest concentration in areas of the body where the skin has had heavy, intermittent exposure to sunlight. Moles are a risk factor for melanoma regardless of skin type. The predisposition to develop few or many moles may be partly hereditary. Most children are born without moles, but some acquire them as they grow older, from about age three on. In a study published in July 1995, Richard Gallagher and his colleagues at the British Columbia Cancer Agency found a direct correlation between a history of childhood sunburns and a high number of acquired nevi in children.[2]

Apparently, the skin forms moles as a reaction to sun exposure. It may even be the case that moles protect sun-damaged melanocytes within them, thus acting as little dark parasols to shade those patches of skin from further assault by the sun. A mole will usually first appear in childhood as a small, flat, tan to dark brown dot the size of a pinhead. It may then slowly enlarge to become a round or oval growth, which may be flat or domed, usually smaller in diameter than a standard pencil eraser. Moles may grow paler as a person matures, and the raised ones often flatten out and eventually disappear late in life.

Some moles have nothing to do with sun exposure. About 1 percent of children have a single mole at birth. These *congenital nevi* are tan to dark brown, flat or slightly raised, and may be greater than a centimeter (nearly half an inch) in diameter. Such moles tend to expand as a person grows and will often sprout hairs. Although some doctors recommend eventual removal of these relatively common congenital nevi to prevent melanoma, the number that develop into melanoma is very small. Of course, parents or children may decide to have the moles removed for cosmetic reasons. Surgical removal is a simple, routine procedure. Another option is to get lifelong monthly inspections of congenital moles, which should be closely watched for changes in color and felt for changes in texture (thickening, for example). It is safe to shave hair associated with some of these moles, and cover-up cosmetics do no harm.

Giant congenital nevi, or *garment nevi*, which cover a significant portion of the body, are fortunately a rare occurrence in children. These moles carry a melanoma risk of 5 to 10 percent, and removal, even by expert plastic surgeons, is very difficult because of their size and depth. Patients with garment nevi require expert consultation and a lifetime of follow-up care, including psychological support.

Although most people have moles that are round and small, about 15 percent of the white population has funny-looking moles, referred to by practitioners as *dysplastic nevi*, or atypical moles. There is some disagreement as to the proper terminology. Dysplastic nevi are different from common moles because they are larger—at least five millimeters across—and either flat throughout or flat with a central dome (like a sunny-side-up egg). They are often variegated—in shades of brown and even pink—and usually have fuzzy, irregular borders. They can even be found on parts of the body that haven't received much sun exposure, such as men's and women's buttocks and women's breasts, as well as on more exposed parts of the body.

You can think about moles in two ways: first as risk markers, and second as potential precursors of melanoma. With regard to risk, the presence of many moles or of a few dysplastic moles makes you two to ten times more likely to get melanoma sometime in your life than the average person with few ordinary moles and no dysplastic moles. Moles tell you that your skin bears watching and warrants protecting.

From another perspective, ordinary moles and dysplastic moles can be precursors of melanoma. In 25 to 30 percent of cases, pathologists examining a melanoma under the microscope see remnants of a preexisting mole. But because there are so many moles out there and relatively few melanomas, the chance that any one mole will become a melanoma is comfortably small. Even in families with a high genetic tendency toward melanoma, the chance that any given dysplastic mole will become a melanoma is estimated at less than one in seven thousand. There are a few melanomas that don't make the usual stops along the tumor progression pathway but become fully fledged without any apparent intervening lesions. One example of truncated evolution is the melanoma that seems to grow from a previously unblemished patch of skin. Another is the nodular melanoma that skips the flat radial growth phase.

When Should a Mole be Removed?

People with many dysplastic nevi often have to have numerous biopsies. Happily, as is true of most colon polyps and breast lumps, most moles that warrant a biopsy are not malignant.

So why not just take off all moles? Just as the prophylactic surgical removal of healthy breasts (that is, surgical removal of healthy tissue as a preventive measure) is an extreme way to prevent breast cancer—and generally considered only for those with a very high genetically determined risk—so is the removal of all dysplastic or normal nevi as a preventive to melanoma, and is not recommended. Many people have too many moles for total removal to be practical, and melanoma may arise in apparently normal skin. Most importantly, though, most moles never act up.

Even though the wholesale removal of moles is overkill, there are times when you should have a mole removed. Here are some instances when you should have them taken off:

- If you have had melanoma and also have a solitary dysplastic nevus, removing moles is a good idea when it is easy and cosmetically acceptable to do so.
- If you have a changing or suspicious mole. Change in a mole is perhaps the earliest and most common warning sign of developing melanoma.

- If either you or your physician is concerned about the "look" of a mole, especially one that appears to be changing or that suddenly appeared.

It is wise for people with dysplastic moles (or an abundance of ordinary moles) to keep a vigilant eye on them and have their physicians perform frequent skin exams to detect melanomas early in their evolution. Whole-body photography is also recommended to keep track of moles.

Is Melanoma Hereditary

A misconception about melanoma (and cancer in general) is that it frequently runs in families and is probably caused by a single mutant gene that can be passed from parents to children (a condition called a germline mutation). In fact, only about one in ten patients with melanoma has a close family member who has also had melanoma, and most such patients did not acquire it through a germline mutation. Nevertheless, an important genetic connection exists. The National Cancer Institute and the University of Pennsylvania's Pigmented Lesion Group have been jointly studying twenty-three melanoma-prone families since 1976 to determine why melanoma clusters occur in families and how melanomas can be detected early on. Studying these families has proved beneficial in gaining further knowledge about dysplastic nevi in general, and in developing effective strategies for early detection and prevention for the 90 percent of the population without genes for melanoma susceptibility.

Doctors strongly suspect that melanoma patients who have two or more close blood relatives—parents, siblings, or children—who have melanoma, come from a family with a strong genetic tendency toward it. Recently, several researchers have implicated a mutant gene called *p16*, or *CDKN2A*, that occurs on the ninth chromosome that regulates cell growth. The gene has been found to be the main cause of inherited high susceptibility to melanoma.[3] For a complete overview and 2014 update of genetics and melanoma, go to http://www.cancer.gov/cancertopics/pdq/genetics/skin/HealthProfessional/page4#Section_165 where there is a compilation of studies presented by the National Cancer Institute.

While the search for genes that underlie a very high risk for melanoma continues, particularly in the relatively few melanoma-prone families, researchers are also identifying genetic changes that only slightly elevate the risk but are very common in the population. For example, a modestly elevated risk of melanoma (about twofold) has been found to come from a gene sometimes associated with red hair and freckles that regulates the kind of melanin that melanocytes produce.

Coming from a family with members who have had melanoma or basal or squamous cell cancers is another factor increasing the risk for melanoma, probably because family members share several critical genes (for sun sensitivity, for example) and were raised in the same environment, rather than because they have a single mutant gene in common.

Family members may have inherited a type of skin that burns easily and never tans. As a child, you and your family may have spent a great deal of time vacationing in sunny locations. It is possible that your parents did not take preventive measures against sun exposure and thereby increased your and your siblings' risk of getting skin cancer.

Is There a Gender-Based Predisposition toward Melanoma?

In the United States, men and women get melanoma at about the same rates, yet in countries such as England and Scotland, women develop melanoma more frequently than men. Whether women in those countries spend more time in the sun than men do is unclear.

Regardless of how likely they are to get melanoma in the first place, women seem to survive longer than men once they have it. The natural assumption is that women's increased chance of survival is due to a hormonal or other protective factor. But epidemiologists also speculate that women are more health conscious and thus notice their melanomas earlier. Women also typically pay more attention to their appearance and notice changes in their skin early on.

Another explanation for their higher survival rate is that in women melanoma generally appears on the arms or legs, whereas the head and trunk are more common sites in men. Melanomas located on the extremities have a better prognosis.

Is Pregnancy a Risk Factor for Melanoma?

Young women often become pregnant and sometimes get melanoma. The concurrence of these events is emotionally charged, and it is easy to believe they are causally related. It is also thought that both moles and the skin (particularly skin of the cheeks and nipples, and the line between the navel and the pubis) tend to darken during pregnancy. Still, despite a certain amount of anecdotal evidence, any connection between pregnancy and melanoma is probably coincidental rather than causal.[4] More likely, the link here is that young women get pregnant and young women get melanoma.

Another scary attribute of melanoma that has metastasized into the body is that it can circulate in the blood and penetrate the placenta to reach the baby. Often, a pregnant woman with disseminated melanoma will be advised to have her placenta checked after delivery by a pathologist. But the placenta is apparently an excellent barrier for protecting the baby, and reported cases of the mother's metastasized melanoma transferring to the baby are very rare, even when the placenta shows evidence of the disease. Most physicians will advise women not to get pregnant for at least two to three years after a diagnosis of a melanoma with a significant risk of metastasis; the risk of recurrence is highest during this time. Another factor is that women may not want to simultaneously face the psychological and physical stresses of caring for a young child while dealing with the prospect or actuality of a recurrent and potentially devastating disease.

Will Taking Oral Contraceptives or Undergoing Hormone Replacement Therapy Increase a Woman's Risk?

Elizabeth Holly, professor of epidemiology and biostatistics at the School of Medicine at the University of California at San Francisco, has pioneered studies on hormones affecting the growth of melanoma. In a 1994 study by Dr. Holly, along with Rosemary Cress, MD and David Ahn, MD examined 452 women aged 25 to 59 who had been diagnosed with superficial spreading melanoma and compared them to a control group of more than 900 women of the same age who did not have melanoma.[5]

The researchers studied all the women to determine whether they were at increased risk for developing melanoma after they had received menopausal hormone replacement therapy or used birth control pills. Although they detected only a statistically insignificant increase in the incidence of melanoma among all the women treated with hormones, they concluded that the benefits of hormone replacement therapy (HRT) in preventing osteoporosis and heart disease, as well in mitigating the symptoms of menopause, should outweigh the concern about the possible increased risk of melanoma. Since that study, hormone replacement therapy is no longer prescribed as a long-term solution for short-term menopausal discomfort because of the high correlation between HRT and breast cancer. The group of authors concluded that there is no reason to advise women who have had melanoma to avoid taking either oral contraceptives or hormone replacement therapy (if the latter is indicated).

Does It Matter Where a Person Lives?

Living close to the equator is associated with a higher incidence of melanoma among whites. According to the World Health Organization, white residents of Queensland, Australia, have the highest rate of melanoma in the world: forty patients per one hundred thousand people. To see the rates differ by state in the U.S., go to: http://www.cdc.gov/cancer/skin/statistics/state.htm which shows a map of all states and their incidence rates.

An interesting exception to this pattern is that rates of melanoma in northern Europe (for example, Sweden and Norway) are generally higher than in southern Europe (for example, France and Italy), even after differences in skin type have been taken into account. Epidemiologists suggest that the sun-seeking behavior of northern Europeans may account for this phenomenon. Because their long, dark winters leave them sun starved, when it is sunny they throw caution (and clothing) to the wind.

Writing this chapter gave me pause to wonder why a melanoma formed on my leg. Although I am a health-conscious person, I had no idea how closely I conformed to the profile of a person at high risk for melanoma. My fair skin is freckled and burns easily—type 2 skin. Although I do not think of myself as a sun worshipper, during the first eight years of my life, I lived in southern Arizona and was an avid swimmer. In addition to that intense sun exposure in childhood, I tanned my legs with a sunlamp in high school. I have no family history of melanoma, but most of my four sisters have had basal cell skin cancers, and most were sun worshippers. I have experienced a squamous cell skin cancer that was easily cured by surgery. But I have been fortunate not to have experienced melanoma again since that day in 1989 when I discovered I had melanoma.

CHAPTER 3

Finding Early Melanoma

*A*ccording to the American Cancer Society statistics for the year 2014:

- About 76,100 new melanomas will be diagnosed (about 43,890 in men and 32,210 in women)
- About 9,710 people are expected to die of melanoma (about 6,470 men and 3,240 women)

The society states that in 1980, the lifetime risk of getting melanoma was 1 in 250; in the year 2014, the risk was estimated to be 1 in 50.[1] Melanoma has a deadly reputation, and in the 1930s, when the mortality rate stood at 75 percent, it was. The current death rate from melanoma has dropped to under 10 percent, proof that early identification of melanoma allows for remarkably effective therapy and that knowledge and advancement in treatments has finally come.

Fortunately, melanoma is visible to the naked eye. It is usually pigmented and begins in the top layer of the skin.

These features differentiate melanoma from the other potentially serious cancers and make it easier to spot and treat early. It is also different from many other cancers in a second respect: we know the carcinogen. Sunlight is a major trigger for the changes in melanocytes, which can later result in melanoma.

Still, although they are easy to recognize early on, many melanomas go unnoticed until the later stages, when they are less likely to be curable. Doctors are getting closer to being able to treat advanced-stage melanoma with specifically targeted new drugs and immunotherapies, yet these new therapies still represent a medical frontier. Along with prevention, early detection is still the best line of defense and should be made a top priority in the battle against melanoma. It is important that we teach the public, primary health care providers, and body care practitioners how to recognize incipient melanoma. Early detection by screening will translate into saving lives at a remarkable low cost.

When Is Melanoma Curable?

Melanoma is nearly always curable when it is completely removed before it develops the capacity to spread. In March 1992, Dr. Guerry and his colleagues found, after following six hundred patients throughout the course of thirteen years, that the one-third of the invasive melanomas caught in the radial growth phase did not metastasize (spread) to the rest of the body. The study also revealed that an early melanoma lesion takes a few years on average to advance to the vertical growth phase, when it might metastasize.[2] Thus, ample opportunity usually exists for early detection. Nevertheless, some early melanomas don't give you that latitude but metastasize more rapidly, especially head and neck melanomas. So it's important not to put off having your doctor check out any suspicious signs you may notice.

The earliest step is melanoma in situ, confined to the epidermis, or the top layer of the skin. Dr. Clark referred to this as the radial growth phase because early melanoma appears as an irregular circular blotch on the skin that gradually expands along the radii of an imperfect circle. The next step in early melanoma is the invasive radial growth phase, called invasive because the melanoma extends shallowly into the dermis, the second layer of the skin. Melanomas treated at either of these steps are essentially 100 percent curable. The following step in the tumor progression is the vertical growth phase, in which a part of the melanoma starts to elevate (become dome shaped) as it grows in and through the underlying dermis. Even at this later stage, the overall cure rate is 70 percent. Still, the sooner melanoma is caught, the better; small melanomas in the vertical growth phase are more likely to be cured than larger ones.

How Do I Find Early Melanoma?

Regular skin examination is crucial to finding early melanoma at its most curable stage, so you should set up a schedule of self-examinations. If you have a personal or family history of melanoma or dysplastic nevi, check yourself monthly and have a dermatologist or physician knowledgeable about melanoma check you frequently, too. The frequency of the doctor's exams should be based on the level of risk. For patients at very high risk, as many as four visits per year may be recommended. Self-examination is crucial as a supplement to professional follow-up. The step-by-step procedure is described in the next section.

Patients have demonstrated that they can spot a significant skin lesion just as readily as a physician if they are educated properly. As Berwick and others report in the *Journal of the National Cancer Institute*, people who regularly check themselves for suspicious skin changes are 44 percent less likely to die of melanoma than those who do not.[3] If you are at a higher-than-average risk, you should examine your skin monthly. Mark the date on the calendar. For women, a good way to remember to do the self-exam is to tie it in with your breast exam or your menstrual period. If you are at average to low risk for melanoma, you can do skin self-exams less frequently, every six months or annually. A partner can help you see such hard-to-examine areas as your back and scalp.

Skin Examination: How to Do It, What to Look For

The following steps encompass the basic procedure for self-examination:

1. Start your skin examination in a brightly lit room. You'll need a handheld flashlight, a full-length mirror, a hand mirror, and two chairs or stools.

2. With your back turned to the full-length mirror, inspect the back of your neck and shoulders. Check your face in the mirror, concentrating on your lips, mouth, and ears (front and back).

3. Examine the palms and backs of your hands, and look between the fingers and under the fingernails. Continue inspecting up the wrists, examining both the front and back of your forearms. Scan all sides of your upper arms, and don't forget to look at underarms.

4. Sit down on one chair, and prop up each leg on the other chair one at a time. Check the front and sides of both legs (thigh to shin), ankles, tops of the feet, between the toes, and under the toenails. Examine the heels and soles of the feet.

5. Using a handheld mirror, focus on the neck, chest, and torso. Women should check the undersides of the breasts, the upper back, and any part of the upper arms not viewed in step 3.

6. Using both mirrors, scan your lower back and buttocks and the backs of both legs.

The "Examine Your Skin" page on the MIF website also provides a two-minute video on how to examine your skin properly. You can see it at http://melanomainternational. org/melanoma-facts/examine-your-skin.

Normal moles are small, flat, or dome-shaped skin blemishes or growths, whereas dysplastic nevi are larger, unusual-looking moles that can be warning signs for an increased risk of getting malignant melanoma. Early melanoma can appear as an irregular, inflamed, or spreading flat mole. To help people know and recognize the look of early melanoma, the "ABCDEs of melanoma" mnemonic was coined to refer to the following characteristics of abnormal moles:

- **Asymmetry**: The growth has an irregular shape in that one half of the pigmented spot doesn't look like the other half.
- **Border irregularity**: The border is irregular or notched, not having the smooth round or oval outline of a normal mole.
- **Color variation**: There is a combination of different hues of tan, brown, dark brown, blue, pink, black, or even white. Normal moles are usually a single color,
- **Diameter**: The mole consists of a pigmented spot that is larger than five to six millimeters and may be clearly growing. As melanomas grow to become larger than ordinary moles, a pigmented spot with a diameter bigger than half a centimeter (or a quarter of an inch) should be scrutinized. Any pigmented spot with a diameter of about a centimeter (three-eighths of an inch) requires evaluation.
- **Elevation**: Some early melanomas are slightly elevated throughout. Any pigmented lesion that quickly elevates throughout or develops a bump should be checked right away. (E can also be for evolution, or change in a lesion.)

The only drawback of the ABCDEs is that they do not emphasize the dynamic quality of many melanomas: they have a tendency to change noticeably over weeks or months.

Change is the key word here and is included in one of the American Cancer Society's original seven warning signs of cancer: "A change in a wart or mole." If you notice a color change—especially darkening within a pigmented spot, an enlargement of a previously stable mole, or the appearance of a new pigmented spot of about half a centimeter in diameter, all of particular concern if you are twenty-five or older—have a dermatologist or physician familiar with melanoma check it out. Don't be afraid or embarrassed to see someone about a skin change.

Professional Skin Examinations

Your family doctor probably won't perform a skin examination unless you have specifically requested it. Many general practitioners don't make skin exams a normal part of a routine physical, nor do they teach self-examination techniques. Because little time is spent in medical school teaching the technique of skin examination, few practitioners are sufficiently skilled in its performance or aware of its importance. Doctors today are already overwhelmed by a battery of required screening tests they have to perform. However, you might be the influencing factor that gets the doctor to start practicing skin examination just by requesting it!

If you are at high risk for melanoma, your first checkup should include a complete skin examination, risk assessment, and discussion of the warning signs of melanoma and the best way to protect yourself and your family from overexposure to the sun.

Digital technology has advanced photography as an educational and prognostic tool. Photographic techniques for tracking melanoma should be used on those people with a high risk, such as those with many dysplastic nevi or many ordinary moles and a family history of melanoma. These folks should have baseline photographs of their skin taken for purposes of comparison on subsequent visits. Photography often prevents unnecessary surgeries and mole removals. Skin may change more during hormonal fluctuations, so the skin should be checked more frequently during pregnancy.

If you are still worried about something on your skin after visiting your doctor, and he hasn't satisfied your concerns, seek another opinion, preferably from a dermatologist. Melanomas can be tricky to diagnose. It's your body, and you should trust your intuition if you think something is wrong. Don't wait for potentially more serious symptoms or signs to arise. Two other features of melanoma are also worth mentioning. Some melanomas look ugly and may give rise to comment. If someone says to you, "What's that? You should get it taken care of!" do something about it. Some melanomas itch or sting persistently. Any pigmented lesion that does should be checked.

Where Do Melanomas Most Often Appear?

Melanomas most commonly appear on the backs of men and women, the chests and abdomens of men, and the legs of women. Surprisingly, melanomas can also occasionally arise in places unexposed to sun, such as the underarms, buttocks, groin, or on or under the breasts in women. Also, in addition to acting directly on the body, the sun may act systemically, and the melanoma may have other causes besides intense sunlight as is the case of mucosal and acral melanoma.

Unfortunately, many people don't realize that something growing on the outside of their body is potentially lethal. Others, by contrast, worry so much about a spot that they go into denial and don't attempt to find out what's wrong. Studies show that people often don't get an early melanoma checked and treated because it grows slowly and doesn't "stick out," or because they haven't experienced any particularly alarming or annoying symptoms, such as the bleeding or ulceration that usually occurs after the melanoma has progressed to a later stage.

A ten-year study of patients with superficial spreading melanoma that was performed at the Pigmented Lesion Clinic and published in the *Journal of General Internal Medicine* finds that people waited an average of nine months to get a lesion checked. A long lag time between diagnosis and treatment can result in a less favorable prognosis. The same study reports that in some cases physicians were responsible for the delay because they didn't recognize the melanoma for what it was or didn't adequately examine the patient's skin.[4] Both of these failures can be blamed on insufficient medical and public health education.

Warning Others

Once you become knowledgeable about the look of melanoma, you may find yourself facing the dilemma of spotting something on strangers that could be melanoma and not knowing how to approach them. A woman in my yoga class had a very obvious melanoma on her upper arm—I could identify it from across the room. I found myself in the awkward position of needing to urge her to get to the doctor quickly without frightening her. I worked with a mutual friend of ours who told the woman's husband of our concern. He applied additional pressure and a month later she had her arm checked by a dermatologist. It was melanoma. Although you may naturally hesitate to approach someone about so personal a matter, you may well save that person's life by speaking up.

Another instance is when I was seated right behind former president George H. W. Bush and his wife, former first lady Barbara Bush, at a cancer meeting. We had met at previous meetings, and they knew my background in melanoma. During the meeting, I noticed a lesion on President Bush's jawline. I studied it for a long time before deciding to say something. It had the features of what I knew to be a suspicious lesion and was camouflaged in a location where it wouldn't be seen easily. During the break, I approached Mrs. Bush with my concerns. Back at the meeting, she told her husband, who immediately turned around and started talking to me about it. He said that he'd had melanoma before and was worried about this particular lesion. He'd had it checked at the Mayo Clinic six months prior but thought it had changed. He wrote me several notes during the meeting. I finally advised him that if he had noticed a change, then he should have the mole checked. He promptly left the meeting and came back a short while later. He said that doctors from Bethesda Naval Hospital were going to meet him at his hotel room later and examine the lesion. That evening, I attended an awards dinner. In the reception line, Mr. Bush pointed me out and said to all in the vicinity, "That woman may have saved my life," and gave me a big hug. I noticed the large Band-Aid on his cheek area where the lesion had been obviously excised by the doctors. A few weeks later, I received an e-mail from the former president reporting that the lesion was benign and thanking me for being "so darned considerate." I had really stuck my neck out and will continue to do so, hoping I'll always be wrong.

Historically, women were the champion melanoma spotters—the most likely to discover their own melanomas—regardless of the anatomical site of the lesion—and those of their partners. One good example of this was a patient I came to know well. Don, an exceptionally bright e-commerce manager with a PhD, noticed a lesion on his leg, covered it with a Band-Aid, and wore shorts. The lesion grew and soon required two Band-Aids to be covered adequately. By then it was itchy and oozing, and he finally had it checked. It was melanoma and had spread to one lymph node. Luckily, he has not had any recurrence of disease. Because this experience taught him the dangerous nature of melanoma, he has helped me educate many others about the potential danger of ignoring a lesion that is changing.

Especially in these days of managed care, when concerns about cost containment make it increasingly difficult for patients to see specialists, it is important for other types of medical professionals who examine the patients more frequently—nurses, nurse-midwives, paramedics, family practitioners, pediatricians, obstetricians and gynecologists, and physical therapists—to be trained to recognize melanoma. Also, nonmedical professionals who tend to people's health and personal care, including hairdressers, massage therapists, lifeguards, and health club personnel, can play an important role in screening.

Are There Any Free Screening Programs for Melanoma?

By contrast with Pap smear screening, which is forty years old, skin cancer screening is relatively new, having been practiced for only about twenty years. Many in the medical profession and government agencies feel that screenings are not cost effective, and they worry that they will be liable in malpractice suits if skin cancer is missed. Although no randomized trial has been done to see how many lives skin cancer screening saves, a recent encounter I had with a melanoma patient at a support group is indicative of the effectiveness of screening. This woman had a mole checked at a skin cancer screening session held at her place of employment. Thanks to the screening, the melanoma was detected in its early stages and she was directed to a dermatologist. She was certain that she would be dealing with something much more serious now if that screening had not been offered, because she would not have had the spot checked otherwise. MIF offers a free skin cancer screening every spring by dermatologists.

Targeting Those at Risk

People who are at higher-than-average risk for melanoma have fair skin that freckles and burns easily, a personal or family history of melanoma or nonmelanoma skin cancers, and many ordinary moles or a few dysplastic moles. But how to target, reach, and motivate the segment of this population is uncertain and is an important research question.

Having found it comfortable and not unduly inconvenient, most people who have been to a screening recommend it to friends and relatives. One of the best features of screening is that it offers an educational moment: the physician or other screener has the opportunity to explain skin cancer prevention practices and skin self-examination while performing the exam.

CHAPTER 4

If You Have Melanoma

*I*t is natural for people to vacillate between compulsion and complacency when it comes to taking care of their bodies. Sometimes when they find something wrong, they put off getting it checked because they think it's probably nothing; or they're so worried it might be something serious, like cancer, that they avoid seeking medical attention altogether. When you spot something suspicious growing on your skin, don't procrastinate—have it checked! Melanoma usually doesn't grow so rapidly that a suspicious growth should be cause for panic, but a biopsy needs to be done expeditiously.

If you are a member of an HMO, as many Americans are, you are probably required to first visit your primary care physician before seeing a specialist for any skin problems. If your primary care physician is judicious and skilled, by all means entrust her with figuring out what the spot you have is. As pointed out before, it is a good idea to ask your doctor to examine your skin thoroughly early on and at appropriate intervals thereafter.

If your primary doctor is concerned about the lesion you point out, she may want to biopsy the growth or refer you to a dermatologist or surgeon for further checks and a biopsy. If your doctor says to watch the skin lesion and come back in six months, insist that it be checked sooner—say, in a month or two—or ask for a referral to a dermatologist. You may run into some resistance now that many health plans restrict the number of referrals to specialists, so be persistent.

What Is the Best Biopsy Procedure?

The pathologist will need to look at a representative specimen to make the diagnosis of melanoma and determine the features that predict its behavior. As a general rule, an *excisional biopsy* is best because it is designed to remove the entire lesion.

This type of biopsy is usually relatively painless. After a local anesthetic is administered, the suspicious spot and a small margin around it are removed, and a few stitches are put in to close the wound. You can resume most activities a few days later.

In certain circumstances, other types of biopsies may be appropriate. If the lesion is small and/or located in a cosmetically sensitive area, such as your face, a *deep-shave biopsy* may be performed. In this procedure, after a local anesthetic is injected, the spot is shaved off with a razor blade. A *punch biopsy* may be used for a very small lesion, and a punch biopsy or an *incisional biopsy* may sometimes be used in the case of a large lesion. In the first technique, all or the most alarming part of the lesion is "punched out" with a cookie cutter-like instrument. In the second, a small portion of the spot is cut out with a scalpel. With either method, disturbance to the appearance of the face, for example, is minimal. The Mohs procedure (developed in 1938 by Dr. Frederic E. Mohs) is sometimes used with melanoma biopsies and definitive removal but is probably better suited for squamous and basal cell cancers. The procedure entails removing a layer of skin at a time to check under the microscope for cancerous cells. If cells still appear, the removal will continue until there is no evidence of cancerous cells. This is done while you are waiting in the procedure room and quite a chunk of skin can be taken. I preferred to have mine closed by a plastic surgeon the following day since it was on a cosmetically sensitive area.

One of the myths about melanoma is that a biopsy will stir up the melanoma cells and cause them to infiltrate the body. No evidence indicates this to be the case. The concern with any biopsy technique other than an excision is that the piece of skin removed will not encompass the entire lesion. Another concern is that taking it out may make it difficult to know the extent to which melanoma has penetrated the skin and consequently determine its stage accurately.

What Questions Should I Ask My Doctor?

Here are some questions to ask about a suspicious skin growth and answers to look for when you see a doctor:

1. *What do you think this growth is?* (Make sure your concern is taken seriously.) Most often, the diagnosis will be something like seborrheic keratosis (a benign lesion) or an ordinary mole.

2. *Are you sure this lesion is benign, and do you think it's sufficient simply to keep an eye on it?* (If the doctor says that no biopsy is necessary.) Ascertain the doctor's degree of comfort with the diagnosis. If the doctor dismisses the growth as nothing worrisome yet you have a gut feeling that it needs to be checked further, get it done.

3. *If you think this might be a melanoma, do you plan to do an excisional biopsy? If not, why?*

4. *When will the results of the biopsy be available?* A week is usually enough time to make a determination.

What Is a Pathology Report?

After the biopsy is completed, the specimen is sent to a *pathologist*—a specially trained physician who interprets the nature of your lesion by examining the biopsy specimen under a microscope. The pathologist's role in proper diagnosis of a pigmented spot is critical: he makes the determination whether it is benign, indeterminate, or malignant, and if it is malignant, what its attributes are. Your doctor will take this information into account in recommending a treatment. That's why it is important to make sure that your biopsy is interpreted by a skilled pathologist.

Your doctor will receive the pathologist's report. If it describes the lesion as suspicious or hard to interpret, you should request that the specimen be reviewed by a *dermato-pathologist*—a specialist in the pathology of the skin—or by a pathologist specializing in melanoma. Such specialized pathologists are often associated with teaching hospitals. Be sure to ask for a copy of your pathology report, even if you don't want to read it. When you ask for it, your physician or the office staff may react with puzzlement. Simply explain that you would like to keep accurate medical records for future reference.

As with any cancer, accurate interpretation of the pathology is crucial in determining proper treatment. The attributes discussed in the pathology report together with your physical examination will usually provide an indication of what surgery is needed, whether you require additional tests and therapy, and will help indicate the likely outcome of the disease. The biopsy report will contain valuable information that you will need later, and if you require a second doctor's opinion, it will speed things up to have the pathology report on hand. Most physicians will also wish to have the glass pathology slides available for review by an expert before offering a second opinion.

Even if you are content with your doctor's diagnosis and treatment plan, it may be a good idea to get a second opinion. Doctors' opinions on treatment and prognosis of melanoma may differ even when they agree on the pathology results. Especially in high-risk situations, going the extra mile is worth the trouble even if you are worn out by worry.

What Questions Should I Ask about the Pathology Report?

When your doctor goes over your pathology report with you, it is best to come prepared with a list of questions.

1. *Who will read the pathology report?* An expert dermatopathologist should probably be on hand if the lesion is difficult to identify or characterize.

2. *What exactly does this pathology mean?* If it is melanoma, the appropriate question would be how do its attributes affect what additional tests I might have and my final prognosis?

3. *What do you recommend as the next course of action?* Be sure to go to the MIF website for definitions of terms used in your pathology report.

A nurse may telephone you to discuss the results instead of the doctor, as often happens when the biopsy shows that the growth is trivial (such as with a seborrheic keratosis or an ordinary mole). If the results are more serious—a nonmelanoma dysplastic mole or melanoma—you should be able to consult personally with your physician. In this case, be prepared to ask if the doctor will be available to discuss the pathology with you.

How Is the Prognosis Determined?

All level 1 and many level 2 melanomas are radial-growth-phase melanomas; the deeper-level melanomas—levels 3, 4, and 5—have almost invariably entered the vertical growth phase. In the early 1970s, Dr. Alexander Breslow of George Washington University Medical School found that it was simpler and more accurate to base a patient's prognosis on the pathologist's measurement (in millimeters) of the thickness of a melanoma that has penetrated below the epidermis than to base it on the numbered level of the melanoma. The numbered level is called Clark's Level and is no longer used by most yet confuses patients into thinking their levels, i.e. I, II, III, IV, are stages of melanoma.

Probably the most current way to predict how patients will do is to first distinguish between radial-growth-phase melanomas (which have essentially no likelihood of recurrence) and vertical-growth-phase melanomas. Further examination of vertical-growth-phase factors allows the physician to better estimate the chance of cure and to decide whether to investigate the nearby lymph nodes.

Dr. Lynn Schuchter and her team at the University of Pennsylvania devised a simplified way of predicting outcomes in melanoma patients. They first examined one hundred reports from different pathologists and found that only half the reports mentioned the thickness of the melanoma or the level of invasion. None of the reports mentioned whether the cancer was still entirely in the radial growth phase. After following 488 patients at the Pigmented Lesion Group for 13.5 years, the team found four independent factors that pathologists and clinicians anywhere could ascertain about patients and their tumor: the patient's age, the patient's sex, the melanoma's thickness, and the melanoma's location. Basing the prognosis on these attributes rather than just thickness reduced the margin of error in predicting survival by 50 percent.[1]

Alternative predictive models now available to clinicians help pinpoint attributes such as the mitotic factor of the tumor. Mitotic count is a measure of how many melanoma cells are dividing. It is often recommended that tumors that are thin and have high mitotic rates be further evaluated with a sentinel-node biopsy. Now that pathologists are reporting more information for use in these improved models, physicians are better equipped to counsel their patients on options for therapy.

What Are the Stages of Melanoma?

After looking at the pathology report, physicians assign a "provisional stage" to a melanoma in order to classify patients according to their chances of being cured, and to guide their choices in further testing and treatment. In general, doctors integrate information on the primary tumor with data on the presence and location of metastases to arrive at the determination of the stage. The following stages are based on the AJCC (American Joint Committee on Cancer) Staging System.

- **Stages I and II**: At these stages, the tumor is confined to the site where it started, and is up to 1.5 millimeters thick. There is no evidence of nearby skin or lymph node involvement or of distant metastasis. The five-year survival rate depends on the melanoma's thickness (and other features) and varies from about 95 percent for people who have stage 1A lesions (a millimeter or less in thickness, not ulcerated, to just under 50 percent for patients with stage 2C lesions (thicker than four millimeters and ulcerated).

- **Stage II**: At this stage, the primary tumor is more than 1.5 millimeters thick and there is no evidence of spreading. The five-year survival rate is about 80 percent. Note that the outcome for patients with stage 1 and 2 disease can be more accurately forecast with the predictive models described earlier.
- **Stage III**: At this point, the melanoma has spread into the nearby skin or, more commonly, into the lymph glands (nodes) near the primary tumor. (The regional nodes for a melanoma on the right forearm, for example, are in the right armpit.) The five-year survival rate depends on the number of nodes involved and whether they have only microscopic amounts of tumor within them or enough of the tumor in them to make the glands big enough to feel by touch (macroscopic involvement). For patients with just one microscopically involved node, the survival rate is as high as 70 percent, while for those with easy-to-feel, enlarged nodes and more than three affected, the survival rate is as low as 15 percent.
- **Stage IV**: When the melanoma has reached this stage, colonies of melanoma cells are present beyond the regional nodes (for example, in the distant skin or nodes, or in the internal organs). The five-year survival rate is currently at 10 percent, but will most likely be raised.

Before you look up your stage and its survival rate, know two things. First, these methods of predicting outcomes, although useful in judging how a group of people will do, are often remarkably inadequate in foretelling your particular future—and many people beat the odds. Second, the current staging system, although an improvement over its predecessor, underestimates in each stage the actual survival. Dr. Guerry and colleagues looked at how well the staging system predicted survival in a large number of patients who are representative of the US population and found that it underestimated survival in each stage by about 10 percent. For example, the AJCC staging system predicts that the ten-year survival rate is 88 percent for a group of patients with stage 1A; in this group the survival rate was actually 97 percent.[2]

The most recent staging update was in 2010 and is discussed here: http://www.skincancer.org/publications/the-melanoma-letter/fall-2010-vol-28-no-3/the-revised-melanoma-staging-system-and-the-impact-of-mitotic-rate

But I expect the staging system may change considerably due to the changing landscape of therapies for melanoma.

What Are Lymph Nodes?

The body's lymphatic system comprises *lymph* (a fluid), *lymph vessels*, and *lymph nodes*. Lymph carries lymphocytes and other cells of the immune system, together with invading bacteria and waste products, through the tissues. It is transported through lymph vessels, the microscopic tubes that carry it into the lymph nodes, little glands that contain millions of immune-system cells. Clusters of lymph nodes are located in strategic places throughout the body. Lymph nodes are an important component of the immune system—the place where immune cells, primarily lymphocytes, are marshaled to fight invading viruses. Thus, the lymph nodes in your neck may swell when your body is trying to fight off an upper respiratory tract infection like a sore throat. Melanoma cells may also travel through lymph vessels into lymph nodes and start reproducing inside them.

If melanoma has spread to your lymph nodes, the disease takes on a different character. Lymph node involvement generally overshadows the pathology of the primary lesion in significance. At this point, melanoma has declared itself as an actual, rather than potential, invader and colonizer. It is exploiting the lymphatic system to colonize new territory. (But please remember that melanoma can also go directly into the blood vessels and bypass the lymph nodes in this area.) Even once melanoma has successfully penetrated the body to reach nearby lymph nodes, the cure rate is considerable. On average, 40–50 percent of those with regional node involvement are cured. (The overall range is 15–70 percent, depending on the number of lymph nodes involved and whether there is microscopic or macroscopic involvement.) If your physician feels an enlarged regional lymph node either on your first visit or on a follow-up, you will probably be advised to have a biopsy taken of the node (by sticking a needle into it to take a sample or by doing an incision to remove the whole node). If melanoma is found, a node dissection will probably be warranted. The three types of dissections are the therapeutic lymph node dissection, elective lymph node dissection, and sentinel lymph node biopsy.

What Is a Lymph Node Dissection?

If melanoma is found in a regional node but nowhere else, you will be advised to have a node dissection; that is, to have the majority of the nodes in that region (for example, the armpit or the groin) surgically removed. (Don't worry; you have plenty of other lymph nodes to take up the slack.) This is called a *therapeutic lymph node dissection.* Some people whose lymph nodes are obviously enlarged by a colony of melanoma cells can be cured by surgery, and a long-standing question has been whether patients whose nodes are not enlarged (but who may be harboring microscopic colonies) might likewise benefit from the removal of regional nodes.

Taking out a group of nodes that are not enlarged is called an *elective,* or *prophylactic, lymph node dissection.* Recent research has made this type of dissection obsolete for two reasons: many or most patients do not gain any benefit from it, and all patients have the potential for side effects such as infections and swelling of the extremities. Patients with pure radial-growth-phase melanomas and most with "thin" lesions (less than a millimeter thick) fall into this category. These patients' melanomas are unlikely to metastasize to the nodes or elsewhere. Patients in whom colonies of melanoma have probably already been established beyond the regional nodes, such as those whose melanomas are more than four millimeters thick and ulcerated, will not benefit from elective dissection either.

What about people with melanomas of intermediate thickness? Couldn't patients who have microscopic colonies in their nodes (still the minority) benefit from node removal before the colonies adapt and propagate elsewhere? This issue is still unresolved. A recent large study of almost 750 patients indicates that among patients under sixty years old, an additional 10 percent with a tumor one to two millimeters thick may survive longer if they have an elective node dissection. Such patients' five-year survival rate is 96 percent, as opposed to 86 percent for those who wait to have nodes removed when and if they become swollen with melanoma. In Australia, where they treat the most cases of melanoma in the world, elective lymph node dissection is no longer routinely practiced and major melanoma units are participating in randomized controlled trials. Their practice dictates that elective lymph node dissection should be considered only for patients younger than sixty years old with primary melanomas on the trunk that are one to four millimeters thick.

What Is a Sentinel Lymph Node Biopsy?

Sentinel lymph node biopsy has become widely used to investigate the regional nodes without removing many or most of them at the outset. It is often straightforward enough to figure out which lymph node group a melanoma is likely to travel to. Melanomas of the leg colonize the nodes in the crease of the groin (inguinal nodes) and arm melanomas wind up in the armpit (axillary nodes).

In other areas—the back, for example—the destination of the cells isn't so obvious. A melanoma of the skin over the right shoulder blade might wind up in the left armpit or the right groin. To find the general destination of such melanomas, physicians have started using a diagnostic technique called *lymphoscintigraphy*. This technique performs a sentinel lymph node biopsy by injecting a small amount of radioactive material around the site of a primary melanoma and then scanning different areas— the armpits and groin, for example—to see which one or ones "light up." The technique was designed to determine whether the lymph nodes that would potentially receive colonies of cells from the primary melanoma have actually done so. Identifying the one or a few sentinel lymph node(s)—the first lymph node(s) poised to receive melanoma colonies—and drawing a sample from them is a refinement to gleaning the information about the melanoma's lymph node drainage and colonization of a group of nodes done by elective lymph node dissection.

In a sentinel lymph node biopsy, the sentinel node is identified by injecting a radioactive solution and/or a blue-colored dye into the spot where the primary melanoma is (or was). This procedure is best carried out prior to the reexcision of the primary melanoma site since a wide reexcision may change the flow of the injected material so that it does not go to the sentinel node. After injecting the dye and waiting half an hour or so for it to reach the node, the surgeon then does the reexcision of the site of the melanoma.

This allows time for the surgeon to identify the location of the lymph node for radioactivity and, with a small incision, locate and remove the "hot" and blue node(s) for a pathology examination. (If after a few days the node is not found to contain melanoma, then it is determined that the adjacent nodes are very unlikely to be involved and no further surgery is necessary. If the sentinel node does reveal melanoma, however, the adjacent nodes are usually removed in what is called a *complete node dissection*, because there are possibly other nodes involved.

What Are the Pros and Cons of Sentinel Lymph Node Biopsy?

The definitive sentinel lymph node biopsy has fulfilled its promise to give both patient and doctor more information more efficiently. Unless the nodes are involved, the patient is spared all but the relatively small incision to check the sentinel node. And it is rare for this procedure to be complicated by such things as infection, swelling of the extremity, or numbness in the region of the incision. Finally, if the doctor determines that the lymph nodes are involved, the patient may be offered nonsurgical adjuvant therapy that has some chance of further cure or prolonging survival.

The decision about what to do after a melanoma has been biopsied and confirmed by the pathologist at this stage when the patient's regional lymph nodes appear normal is more difficult. Some melanoma specialists believe that lymph node mapping and sentinel-node sampling should be done in all patients whose melanomas have any likelihood of metastasizing (for example, patients with lesions with Breslow Level of one millimeter or deeper or lower level with a mitotic factor above 1) Because the procedure is safe and effective, at least in terms of helping to judge the prognosis and directing therapy, most other specialists no longer counsel patients to watch and wait. Mapping and harvesting has become standard practice for melanomas that appear to be at a stage above 1A (melanomas that are one millimeter or less in thickness, are not level 4 or 5, and that are not ulcerated).

Currently, there are experimental trials of the indications and effectiveness of this technique. These trials seek to answer which patients are the best candidates for the procedure and whether taking out nodes that turn out to have melanoma in them prolongs survival and increases the cure rate. Sentinel lymph node biopsy pioneer Donald Morton, MD, and colleagues evaluated the outcomes in 2,001 patients and found that this type of biopsy provides important prognostic information for those with intermediately thick melanomas. They also identified patients having metastasis in their nodes who might benefit from immediate complete removal of the lymph nodes in that region.[3]

What Questions Should I Ask about Regional Lymph Node Involvement?

When you visit your doctor for an assessment, the following questions are useful for discussing regional lymph node involvement:

1. *Can you feel swollen or enlarged regional lymph nodes? If so, how do you intend to investigate them further?*
2. *Do you plan to do lymph node mapping and sentinel lymph node sampling?*
3. *Might I need to have surgery to remove a group of lymph nodes (a lymph node dissection)? If so, what are the side effects? Will there be any numbness or swelling associated with the surgery?*
4. *If I need surgery, will this be an outpatient, same-day, or overnight hospital procedure?*

If I have a node dissection, will it require that a drain be inserted?

5. *For about how long?*
6. *When will the pathology report be available?*
7. *What symptoms should I call you about?*
8. *What should I take for pain after surgery over the next few days?*

Surgery for Your Primary Melanoma

In 1907, Scottish physician William Handley made recommendations that established the style of surgical treatment of melanoma for the fifty years that followed. From the autopsy findings on a single melanoma patient, he concluded that melanomas regularly penetrate the skin around them and fill the tiny lymphatic vessels. He therefore advocated making a wide local excision, about ten centimeters (around four inches) across. The skin graft to close the surgical wound in this procedure left a troublesome scar. Luckily for melanoma patients today, Handley's recommendations have been discredited by studies of many patients over the years. Narrower excisions are now made and lymph node dissection is not performed without compelling reason.

Very wide excisions are still practiced, especially for thick melanomas, but the decision to make a really big excision is based on dogma, as no one has proven that anything beyond a relatively narrow excision improves survival. Local recurrence of all but the thickest melanomas is rare following narrow excisions, and is almost never the cause of disseminated disease. Death from melanoma usually occurs as a result of microscopic cells traveling even before the primary melanoma is excised from the lymph nodes and other organs. (Your primary melanoma is the first place on your body it is found, usually in a skin lesion.)

Before the definitive surgery is performed, diagnostic tests such as chest X-rays and bloodwork are often done in addition to the physical exam, except when the melanoma is very thin (e.g., in stage 1A), depending on the doctor's viewpoint. An MRI or CAT or PET scan may also be done if the less technical workup shows something suspicious or if you are part of a study that requires these. A PET scan pictures the accumulation in the body of a radioactive form of glucose after it is injected in a vein. Many tumors, including melanomas, and areas of inflammation (e.g., abscesses) produce positive scans. The role of this test in taking care of patients with melanoma is still being worked out. What is clear is that it does not need to be done in people with low and intermediate stages of disease, including those with microscopic involvement of regional nodes.

What Should I Look for in a Surgeon?

The mindsets of surgeon and patient will have an important bearing on the details of your surgery. Some guidelines on the possible scope of the operation follow, but you should pick a surgeon who will pay attention to achieving satisfactory cosmetic results and who will discuss in detail what to do about lymph nodes and follow-up after surgery. A dermatologist will sometimes handle the initial biopsy and the smaller surgeries, or you may be referred to a general surgeon or plastic surgeon for larger lesions, and certainly to a specialist if the melanoma is in a cosmetically important place like the face. Be sure to interview a few surgeons to understand their specific talents and experience with melanoma. You may find a surgical oncologist who specializes in melanoma or other cancers. The larger the lesion, the more complex the surgery in most instances and the more specialized the surgeon should be. You should consider going to a medical center with expertise in melanoma, particularly if it has a practice that arranges for you to see all physicians who might be involved in your care during one visit—dermatologist, surgeon, oncologist, psychologist, and medical photographer, for instance.

How Big Will the Surgical Wound Be?

Melanomas in the radial growth phase, whether in situ or invasive, are generally treated by taking off a band of skin and subcutaneous tissue half a centimeter to one centimeter in width. (The smallest distance from the melanoma or the scar at the biopsy site to where the surgeon cuts is called the margin.) Thin melanomas in the vertical growth phase (those less than a millimeter thick) can safely be treated by taking off one-centimeter margins. Melanomas that are one to two millimeters thick usually require removing one- to two-centimeter margins. For those that are over two milli-meters thick, two centimeters margins are usually removed; sometimes the margins are wider for the thick lesions (of over four millimeters) and for those in which the pathologist sees evidence of growth into small skin nerves (something called neurotropism). Even with a two-centimeter margin, only a small percentage of patients will need a skin graft, which can be troublesome cosmetically. For melanomas exceeding four millimeters, some doctors recommend excising a margin of three centimeters or greater.

What to Ask the Surgeon

Before scheduling the surgery, you'll want to ask the surgeon a few questions:

1. *What will my surgery be like—how big a deal will it be?*
2. *Do you regularly treat people with melanoma?*
3. *What margin will you aim for?* You might ask your sur-geon to draw the boundaries of the excision on your skin with a pen so that there won't be any surprises when you see it after surgery.
4. *Will I need a skin graft? What part of my body will the graft come from?* Often the graft is taken from the buttocks or thighs.

5. *How long will I be incapacitated?*
6. *Will I be an inpatient or outpatient? If an inpatient, how long will I have to stay in the hospital?*
7. *Will I have general anesthesia? Is local or regional anesthesia possible?*
8. *What about postoperative pain?*

What Happens After Surgery?

After you have been told the stage of your disease based on the pathology reports and the surgery is complete, a schedule for follow-up examinations and diagnostic tests will be set up for you. Follow-up guidelines will differ from doctor to doctor and are based in part on the stage of your melanoma and recognition that the first three years after therapy are the time of highest risk of relapse.

As an example, here is what the Pigmented Lesion Group does for melanoma follow-up: it divides melanoma patients into two groups—(1) those with low-risk lesions, pure radial-growth-phase melanomas, and stage 1A lesions; and (2) those with higher-risk disease, including patients who have thicker primary lesions, patients who have vertical-growth-phase melanomas, and patients whose melanomas have metastasized to nearby skin or regional lymph nodes.

The low-risk group, whose melanomas are in the radial growth phase and are thin in Breslow Level, will be checked every six months for two years, and yearly thereafter. Because it is highly improbable that melanoma in the radial growth phase will metastasize for these patients, the follow-up consists only of an exam to determine their physical status. During the exam, the doctor is on the lookout not only for recurrence of melanoma at the surgery site or in the regional lymph node, but also for the possible development of a second, new primary melanoma, which should be readily curable if it is caught early on.

Patients in the highest risk group (for example, those with an ulcerated melanoma thicker than four millimeters), with treated tumors in the vertical growth phase or treated metastases of the lymph nodes or skin between the primary site and the nearest lymph nodes, are seen every three months for the first year after surgery and every four months for the second and third years. During the fourth through fifth years, visits are scheduled every six months. From the sixth year on, visits are annual. These patients are advised to have a chest X-ray at every other visit for the first three years. Thereafter, X-rays are done yearly. If during that time something new shows up, such as melanoma in a lymph node, the physician reverts to examining the patient on the original schedule.

Referral to an Oncologist

If any of the nodes are found to be positive from the sentinel-node biopsy, and/or your lesion has features that make it high risk, you will most likely be referred to a medical oncologist to determine future treatment. It is recommended that you choose an oncologist who is familiar with melanoma and has treated many other melanoma patients. Make sure you are on the same page as the oncologist regarding the type of treatment plan you prefer. You must weigh quality-of-life issues against the toxicity and side effects of the several adjuvant therapies available. Adjuvant therapies are those that will potentially serve as an additional therapy to surgery. Sometimes performing radiation therapy on the region where macroscopic nodes were removed is considered. More often, a kind of therapy that works throughout the body will be offered as an option; for example, the immune-system hormone Intron A (interferon alfa-2). Remember that no therapy other than surgery has yet been proven to increase the rate of overall survival. Therefore, a real choice you can make with your doctor is to watch and wait; for stage III patients this may be an especially viable option.

Questions to Ask the Oncologist

When you visit the oncologist, you will want to ask the following questions:

1. *How many lymph nodes are involved? What is the prognosis of a group of patients like me?* (No doctor can tell you what your fate is.)
2. *Did you check my tumor for* BRAF *status?*
3. *What is the risk the melanoma has spread to other parts of the body?*
4. *What additional treatment do you suggest?*
5. *Do you know of any clinical trials that might be promising?*
6. *Will you help me find and enroll in a clinical trial?*
7. *Do I need specialized scans? How often?*

8. *Will you work with me if I choose no further treatment? Or if my disease gets to the point that I need only excellent palliative care?*

How Do I Perform a Lymph Node Self-Exam?

You can keep an eye on your own lymph nodes, as well as on your skin, to observe any changes. Every month or so, check the lymph node nearest to where your melanoma occurred. My melanoma was on my lower leg, so I would check the crease where the thigh joins the trunk or body to make sure I did not have a firm lump bigger than the width of a thumbnail. If the melanoma is on your head or in the trunk area, it is a little trickier to figure out which lymph nodes might be involved. It is normal to feel small lymph nodes up and down your body.

Ask your doctor exactly what to look for when you examine your lymph nodes. Dr. Guerry cautions that because "there are no absolutes in medicine, we also let people know that even with thin melanomas, they run a tiny chance of a metastasis and that we and they and their physicians ought to keep an eye (or hand) on the lymph nodes."

In 1989, I certainly didn't know whether I would be among the fortunate 95 percent who were cured or the unlucky 5 percent who weren't. The first doctor I saw told me that I had a 20 percent chance of recurrence. I am now checked only once a year for any skin changes or lymph node involvement and so far no recurrence has appeared.

Where Can I Get More Information About Melanoma Treatments? (And a Word of Caution about the Internet)

A diagnosis of melanoma may throw you and your family into a tailspin. You may want to have all the information you can get your hands on, and that is a good thing. But always be cautious about what you read. The news is full of sensationalist reports of new "cures" for cancer—when you read the fine print, you find out that the study was done on mice and has only a slight chance of working on humans, or it worked in only a small group of people, or that the study was financed by the pharmaceutical company that manufactures the agent.

And then there's information you get from the Internet, which has opened up a whole new world of medical information instantly at your fingertips. Beware of chat groups and bulletin boards, as they are not typically reviewed by anyone with melanoma expertise and are primarily based on personal stories that may have nothing to do with yours. Patients' opinions are often expressed that may not reflect the lessons learned from careful study/interpretation of studies, which is what your oncologist and her colleagues should be able to provide. A study of melanoma information on the Internet was published in the *Journal of Clinical Oncology* that finds inaccuracies in 14 percent of the sites with information on cancer.[4] It was also found that many legitimate sites didn't come up in the researchers' initial web search because ample funding may be the criteria to get top billing with the search engines. You should ask your health care provider which sites are accurate, and bring up information that you'd like verified.

The Health on the Net (HON) Foundation, is a Swiss non-profit dedicated to verifying the reliability of health-oriented websites by issuing a HONcode designation for those sites that meet their code of conduct. According to their website, "HON was founded to encourage the dissemination of quality health information for patients and professionals and the general public, and to facilitate access to the latest and most relevant medical data through the use of the Internet." The MIF is proud to have earned HONCode approval. Please see more, including patient tips for searching the Internet for reliable information at www.healthonnet.org.

CHAPTER 5

When Melanoma Metastasizes

*M*elanomas, particularly thick ones, can cast spin-offs through the lymph vessels and bloodstream to other parts of the body. Although doctors can sometimes predict which melanomas are likely to spread, and can make educated guesses about the timing and pattern of spread, the disease can show up in a variety of places in the body according to its own timetable.

What should be done if melanoma spreads? The answer depends on the patient, the tumor, and the treatments that are currently considered promising. Because clinical researchers are constantly exploring new therapies to fight melanoma, you will want to get in touch with the resources listed on MIF's website, http://melanomainternational.org/

web-resources, to learn about the centers that offer current research and therapies. They are listed by state and the links take you directly to the melanoma programs at the centers. International patients can find global centers listed by country at http://melanomainternational.org/web-resources/global-resources.

Finding the Right Doctor

The first step toward taking care of your metastasized melanoma is choosing a doctor in whom you feel a high level of confidence. You might be fortunate enough to find a physician in your community who is knowledgeable about melanoma, although there are few specialists in the field. If not, it is worth the trouble to travel a certain distance to find the right doctor. A physician who deals with melanoma on a regular basis (and even better, one that is working on melanoma research) will probably be better informed about treatments and more relaxed in talking to you about the disease. Melanoma specialists are frequently able to link up with a qualified network of surgeons, pathologists, oncologists, and mental health professionals, and thus provide you with more comprehensive care. It might be a good idea to go for your initial evaluation and surgery at a specialized clinic no matter the location, as long as you can get there, and then have your follow-up checkups locally. MIF provides travel scholarships for patients to travel to leading melanoma centers for clinical trials and second opinions. You can apply and find out more at http://melanomainternational.org/who-we-are/ patient-access-grants-apply.

Needless to say, your doctor's professional expertise will be critical. The practitioner's personality may also matter to you, although it does not necessarily give an assurance of medical proficiency. You will probably be able to gauge the doctor's willingness to give you a say in your own treatment and treat you like a respected colleague as you work together. Where do you find a doctor who will cooperate with you in this way? A teaching hospital will usually have a good melanoma team. A hospital that has been designated a Comprehensive Cancer Center by the National Cancer Institute offers additional advantages because it has demonstrated that it has a strong research program that supports its clinical practice in most instances. When looking for a doctor, call ahead and talk with the nursing staff. You can often get a feel from the initial contact for how the clinic or practice operates. Nurses are also an excellent resource—they may be able to recommend a good doctor, and their knowledge is based not only on medical expertise but on being a physician's coworker. You might also ask other patients for their recommendation. You can do so on MIF's forum, www.melanomaforum.org, and find out what other patients recommend.

What Is Metastasis?

Metastasis is both a process and a thing. It is the process by which cancer spreads from its starting point in the primary tumor to other parts of the body. It occurs when cancer reproduces and sheds cells through the lymphatic system and blood vessels. The word is also used to refer to a single secondary lesion or the existence of the metastatic process.

Whether and where these cells are able to grow can be explained by the soil and seed theory, so named because of the parallels between melanoma cells and seeds, both of which can take root far from the parent. Melanomas grow on receptive terrain. If a melanoma cell is delivered, for example, to a lymph node (fertile ground), it may, after a variable period of dormancy, sprout into a colony of cancerous cells (a metastasis). This colony may in turn generate new ones. Thus, the word metastasis is also used to refer to an actual collection of malignant cells that are in a place away from the original or primary tumor site. These cells might be felt as an enlarged lymph node or seen as a round shadow on a chest X-ray or CAT or PET scan. A metastasis can be thought of as a collection of many cells, descendants of the first seeds cast from the primary tumor that form a mass at another site. Metastases sometimes manifest themselves as palpable lumps in the skin or lymph nodes, or they may occur and grow within an internal organ and cause it to malfunction.

Two Types of Metastases

Melanoma metastases fall into two general categories. *Regional metastases*, the first category, are confined to the region of the primary tumor. This region encompasses the nearby lymph nodes and the expanse of skin between the primary site and those lymph nodes. Regional metastases are thought to be established by seed cells that travel from the primary site via tiny lymph vessels.

Distant metastases, the second category of metastatic disease, develop beyond the region of the primary melanoma; that is, they are caused by cells disseminated far from the primary site itself, the skin around it, and the regional lymph nodes. Common destinations for melanoma cells include nonregional skin and lymph nodes, the lungs, liver, and brain. Melanoma cells spread after first entering small blood vessels at the primary site or in the regional lymph nodes.

Treatments for Regional Metastases

Metastases confined to skin in the region of the primary site are usually surgically removed. Equivalent techniques are sometimes used, including laser surgery (to vaporize certain surface metastases) and the injection of inflammatory, immune-stimulating agents. In the case of multiple metastases in the skin and subcutaneous tissue of an extremity, the whole limb may be treated through *regional perfusion*. During this procedure, a tourniquet is applied to isolate the blood supply of the limb from the rest of the blood's circulation. The diseased arm or leg is then infused with heated cancer-killing drugs. The agents are injected into the artery supplying the limb and are then removed through the vein. Regional perfusion, by treating only the affected limb, avoids the systemic toxicity of the drugs. Unfortunately, it will not take care of melanoma

cells that have migrated elsewhere in the body. The procedure, which must be performed by a specially trained surgical oncologist, requires general anesthesia and several days
of hospitalization.

Intralesional Therapies

There are a few therapies that are injected directly into
lesions (subcutaneous intransit metastasis), known as *intralesional therapies*, where there has been some reported bystander
effect to systemic disease. Although still early in clinical trial,
two being studied are talimogene laherparepvec (T-VEC), a
type of herpes simplex virus; and PV-10, a 10 percent solution
of the rose bengal dye. Further study of both should yield
results of the efficacy for future use. The combination of
these agents, and others, with systemic agents such as immunotherapies and *BRAF* could lead to interesting developments
in melanoma treatment strategies.

Adjuvant Therapy

Adjuvant therapy is any treatment intended to supplement
the surgical removal of cancer. Adjuvant radiation therapy
is sometimes used where many lymph nodes are involved in
the melanoma, or where the disease is growing through the
nodes into the surrounding tissue. Generally, however, adjuvant therapy is given in a way that affects the whole body: it
is designed to kill components of the disease that may have
escaped to other parts of the body before the primary tumor
or diseased lymph node is removed. Doctors call on adjuvant

therapy when the disease is statistically likely to have metasta-sized, but no evidence of distant disease is actually uncovered even when the patient is scanned from head to toe. Adjuvant therapy is usually recommended for: thick melanomas (where lymph nodes are involved) and where there is no lymph node involvement, or stage II disease; or for stage III disease with lymph node involvement.

When the risk of discovering subsequent metastasis is high, two precautionary steps can be taken. First, the surgeon can remove the primary lesion and sometimes the regional lymph nodes. Next, a doctor, usually a medical oncologist, can administer an adjuvant agent with the aim of killing any melanoma cells remaining elsewhere—ideally, preventing the disease from ever returning. Applying adjuvant therapy is like putting preemergent weed killer on a garden.

Just as with breast cancer, where a lumpectomy and radia-tion are followed by chemotherapy and hormonal therapy to increase the probability of a complete cure, some melano-mas are treated with surgery followed by adjuvant therapy. But unlike breast cancer, it has been difficult with melanoma to find a treatment that will kill undetectable metastases. Figuring out who is most likely to benefit from effective adju-vant therapy has been relatively straightforward: it includes people whose melanomas are thicker than four millime-ters, particularly if the tumor is ulcerated, and those whose regional lymph nodes are involved (especially when they are several or macroscopic nodes). The problem has been find-ing a therapy that works.

Interferon Alfa-2b, Sold as Intron A

Interferon alfa-2b, sold as the pharmaceutical Intron A, is a biotechnically synthesized protein that is identical to a protein the body produces when it fights off viral infections. Interferon alfa-2b is the only agent currently approved by the U.S.Food and Drug Administration (as of 2014) as adjuvant therapy for melanoma patients. The approval was based on a clinical research study, published in the January 1996 issue of the *Journal of Clinical Oncology*, in which patients with thick melanomas or regional lymph node involvement received either high doses of the interferon or no adjuvant therapy. The highest doses were given intravenously for a month, and then lower doses were self-administered as a skin injection three times a week for eleven months. Five years later, 46 percent of the patients treated with the interferon were still alive, as opposed to only 37 percent of the untreated patients.[1] Subsequent studies have confirmed interferon alfa-2b's ability to delay the appearance of metastatic disease by a year on average, but have called into question its ability to prolong survival.[2] Because of this factor and the continuing dialog on the efficacy of the interferon, the FDA's Oncology Drug Advisory Council decided in 2002 that researchers would not be required to use interferon as the control arm in clinical trials of treatments for melanoma.[3]

When given in the high doses that are apparently necessary to effectively delay the growth of melanoma cells,

interferon alfa-2b has many side effects. Patients taking it feel at first as though they have a bad case of the flu. This effect wears off with time and can be alleviated with other medicines. Interferon alfa-2b may also cause a range of bad reactions, including severe toxic damage to the liver, significant decreases in blood counts, hair loss, fertility dysfunction, and neuropsychological reactions such as severe, significant depression. These side effects are certainly troublesome, but they can be ameliorated by decreasing the dose of interferon, taking holidays from it, and using other medications to combat its symptoms (including acetaminophen for the flu symptoms, antidepressants for depression). As difficult as this therapy can be, it is worth it for some; a quality-of-life analysis indicates that, in general, a higher quality of life was gained from the delay of disease recurrence than was lost from negative side effects. If the patient is concerned about future fertility, they should discuss whether this drug is for them.

A one-year course of interferon alfa-2b (the recommended duration) costs anywhere from $30,000 to $68,000 for the interferon alone. Additional costs may be incurred for medications to control the many side effects. The first twenty doses are given intravenously in a doctor's office five days a week for a month. Blood tests need to be performed frequently. Medical insurance should pay for the interferon as well as the other expenses incurred but don't assume this. You will need to discuss with your doctor, the best being a medical or surgical oncologist, whether interferon alfa-2b is the right drug for you. Many of the top melanoma research centers no longer

prescribe interferon and note that close observation of the patient along with regular checkups provide the same overall survival benefit.

What about Biochemotherapy?

Sometimes used as an adjuvant therapy for stage III and traditional therapy for stage IV, *biochemotherapy* uses a combination of chemotherapy, interferon alfa-2b, and IL-2 or interleuken 2, plus other agents. It requires patients to be hospitalized for treatment and often causes them to experience blood, gastro, and potential cardiovascular toxicities. In a study published in *Current Oncology*, Verma and colleagues looked at nine randomized controlled trials of biochemotherapy and found that none of the studies produced a statistically significant survival improvement for patients.[4]

Are Other Adjuvant Therapies Available?

Sargramostim (marketed under the trade name Leukine) is a recombinant granulocyte macrophage colony-stimulating factor (also known as GM-CSF), and was once a promising adjuvant stage III therapy, but its effectiveness was disproved in final clinical trials. It is still is being discussed and studied in combination therapy and in clinical trials for stage IV.

Quite a number of adjuvant therapies are undergoing preliminary exploration or clinical trial. Many are less toxic than interferon alfa-2b and will probably be approved by the FDA. The difficulty lies in proving whether an agent works with stage III disease, as often there is no measurable disease

(tumor size), as there is in stage IV disease, to compare after administering the drug. Nevertheless, adjuvant therapy for stage III disease is an unmet need. Newly approved drugs, Yervoy and the PD-1 immunotherapies, and *BRAF* therapies are in clinical trial for stage III adjuvant therapy. Be sure to check for updates on the clinical trials discussed on MIF's melanomaforum.org as well as the listing by the National Cancer Institute at www.clinicaltrials.gov to find information on clinical trials for your stage of disease and programs in your geographical area.

Treatments for Disseminated Melanoma

Melanoma that appears throughout the skin or has spread to the internal organs is difficult to treat in the vast majority of cases. While some patients have lasting responses to therapy, some do not. New therapies in the past three years have brought considerable promise to achieving lasting remission. The therapeutic plan for an individual patient will depend on prior treatment; the location and extent of the metastatic disease; the patient's age, general health, and personal wishes; and the availability of clinical research studies on new kinds of therapy

Chemotherapy and Biological Therapies

Although *chemotherapy* sometimes produces regression of disseminated melanoma, it only rarely results in long-term survival. Chemotherapy for melanoma patients has shown only minor response over the years. Several kinds of chemotherapy drugs are still used alone or in combination. DTIC,

the proprietary name of dacarbazine, is a drug approved by the FDA for melanoma and has long been used intravenously and as a comparator in clinical trials. The pharmaceuticals Temodar, Temodal, and Temcad, versions of temozolomide, are taken by mouth and are chemically related to DTIC. Although not substantiated in scientific research, temozolomide is still thought by some clinicians to cross the blood-brain barrier to combat brain metastases. This chemotherapy has not been proven as an effective treatment for melanoma patients.

Biological therapies—for example, vaccines and immunological hormones called cytokines—are still offered for melanoma treatment. An FDA-approved treatment for patients with stage IV melanoma is the cytokine interleukin-2 (IL-2). Although 94 percent of patients do not get a promising result from the drug, 6 percent have been documented to have lasting remissions after treatment with interleukin-2. Dr. Stephen Rosenberg of the National Cancer Institute has pioneered the use of this drug alone and in combination with methods of triggering the immune system to attack melanoma. Current research is trying to uncover the mechanisms by which IL-2 works and supplement it with other therapies. Because IL-2 therapy is quite toxic when given in its most effective (high) doses, it is given over about a week in the hospital.

Molecularly Targeted, or *BRAF* Therapy

A new way of conceptualizing and approaching cancer therapy is based on a deep understanding of the circuitry of cancer

cells and how it has been broken to enable the malignant cells to divide, invade, spread, and colonize other tissues. The aim of this approach is to find medicines that will specifically interfere with abnormal signaling within cancer cells, referred to as *molecularly targeted therapy*.[5] A clue that researchers use to pinpoint what drives abnormal signaling is the discovery of a gene or genes that have commonly been mutated in a particular malignancy. Certain more active mutations "turn on" a protein, while others disable the function of the protein that the gene encodes. These activating mutations are particularly sought as potential therapeutic targets. More than a decade ago, a study of the genome in a number of malignancies found that about 50 percent of melanomas are correlated with a mutation in the *BRAF* gene, a member of a family of so-called *RAF kinase* genes. The mutation causes the *BRAF* gene to make a protein that is inappropriately turned on to activate a particular signaling pathway that stimulates cell growth and helps it avoid death.

When you are diagnosed with melanoma, your oncologist should bring up the term *BRAF* with you when discussing therapies. For *BRAF*-targeted therapies to be considered, testing of melanoma tissue for the presence or absence of a *BRAF* mutation is required. Please note, this is not a genetic mutation of you, but of the tumor. If you qualify, there may be opportunities to get this therapy or participate in clinical trials with *BRAF*-targeted therapies, which have been shown to extend progression-free and overall survival by tumor reduction. These drugs may be given alone or in combination with

other drugs. Zelboraf, one of the *BRAF* therapies, received early FDA approval. More recently approved, Dabrafenib and Mekinist (a MEK inhibitor) can be given as a combination therapy or Dabrafenib can be given alone. Other *BRAF* and MEK agents or inhibitors that block the MEK protein are in trials and may be marketed in the near future.

The testing done to determine if your tumor is positive for the *BRAF* mutation will seek to find out if you have the most common alteration in the *BRAF* gene, the V600E mutation. Currently, testing for this mutation takes place at most university-based pathology labs and involves the cobas HPV test as well as numerous other tests.

The interaction between the *BRAF* gene and protein is not an easy concept to explain. The *BRAF* gene makes a protein called B-raf, which is involved in sending signals on pathways in cells that contribute to cell growth. It is found in normal cellular-growth activity. When it is overactive, it can lead to excessive cell growth and cancer. Among other proteins involved in the cell-signaling pathway, B-raf is the most prominent one researchers have looked at.

A gene may become mutated in many types of cancer. In melanoma, the *BRAF* gene is commonly mutated, which causes a change in the B-raf protein. A mutated *BRAF* gene accelerates tumor cell growth, and this change can increase the growth and spread of cancer cells. Therefore, *BRAF* drugs target the cancer-causing mutation in melanoma. About 50 percent of melanoma patients have this mutation. Interestingly enough, this *BRAF* mutation is also seen in

benign moles. *BRAF* mutations are largely restricted to melanomas that arise from sun-exposed skin, and rarely from acral, ocular, or mucosal types of melanoma, whose origin is not yet clearly known.

These new *BRAF*-targeted therapies are administered as oral capsules. They are intended to inhibit the B-raf protein from potential tumor growth and activity. A B-raf inhibitor selectively binds to and inhibits the activity of B-raf, which in turn may inhibit the proliferation of tumor cells that contain a mutated *BRAF* gene. Some people refer to these therapies simply as anti-*BRAF*. Side effects of the drug include rash, fever, sun sensitivity, gastrointestinal disturbance, and fatigue. If the reactions are severe, the patient may be given lower doses or taken off of the drug entirely.

MEK inhibitors have demonstrated positive effects in patients whose melanomas harbor *BRAF* mutations. MEK uses the enzyme activated by *BRAF*, so MEK inhibitors are thought to exert a similar effect as *BRAF* inhibitors. However, recent evidence suggests that MEK inhibitors can complement the effect of *BRAF* inhibitors. A combination of *BRAF* and MEK inhibitors has demonstrated improvements in initial response as well as durability of response, and the combination has been approved by the FDA. There is also extensive laboratory evidence and preliminary clinical evidence that MEK inhibitors may be useful in some patients whose melanomas do not have a *BRAF* mutation, but have other genetic alterations that activate the same signaling pathway. In particular, mutations in the *NRAS* gene appear to have at least

partial sensitivity to MEK inhibitor therapy. Several clinical trials are ongoing to test MEK inhibitors alone and in combination with other targeted therapies. MEK inhibitors have a distinct side effect profile compared to *BRAF* inhibitors: they cause an acne-like rash, diarrhea, fatigue, and visual changes. The C-Kit mutation sometimes found in mucosal melanoma is also being studied for therapeutic solutions.

Immunotherapies

It is well known that melanoma is an immune-responsive disease, which explains some cases where the disease disappears on its own.[6] Deciphering the code to turn on the body's immune system to effectively eliminate melanoma tumors, however, remained elusive until recently. The older immunotherapies IL-2 and interferon, although still in use, may be toxic to the whole body and pan out to be ineffective for the majority of patients.

Immunotherapy is a type of cancer treatment that uses the body's immune system to ward off the creation of tumors and destroy those already formed by malignant melanoma tumor cells. This type of therapy stimulates the immune system with highly purified proteins or molecules that help it do its job more effectively. The immune system is a network of cells and organs that work together to defend the body against foreign substances (antigens), such as bacteria, virus, or tumor cell. When the body discovers such a substance, several kinds of cells (T cells) go into action as an immune response.

Scientific advances have led to an improved understanding of the interactions between the immune system and tumors, generating renewed interest in this method of melanoma treatment. Indeed, there have been recent FDA approvals of immunologic agents, and there are many ongoing trials of novel immunotherapies in melanoma.

The safety and efficacy of these new agents has much improved the outlook for immunotherapy treatments for melanoma. The first type of immunotherapy, an anti-CTLA-4 antibody called ipilimumab (commonly called IPI), commercially manufactured as Yervoy, was approved by the FDA in March 2011 to treat patients with stage IV melanoma that has spread or cannot be removed by surgery. IPI is a monoclonal antibody that works by activating the immune system through targeting a molecular brake, called CTLA-4, which immune cells use to prevent hyperactivation of the immune system. IPI blocks the inhibitory signal so that cancer cells can be recognized and destroyed by immune cells more effectively. On February 1, 2012, Canada approved Yervoy for treatment of unresectable, or metastatic, melanoma in patients who fail, do not have a favorable response to, or do not tolerate other systemic therapy for advanced disease. Additionally, in November 2012 Yervoy was approved in the European Union (EU) for second-line treatment of metastatic melanoma, and in July 2013 it was approved in Australia for reimbursement by the health authority.

Patients' response rate is estimated to be between 15 and 20 percent, and there are reported cases of long-term

response. It can take as long as twenty-three weeks to kick in. Four doses of Yervoy are given intravenously for ninety minutes every three weeks. The cost of the drug is approximately $120,000 for the course of treatment. The side effect profile includes symptoms of diarrhea that can develop into colitis, rash and/or dermatitis, and endocrine gland malfunction. Some people have mild side effects, while others have to discontinue the immunotherapy when symptoms become severe and/or the disease progresses while on the drug.

The introduction of medicines that block another immune-system brake called PD-1 brings more optimism to therapy options for melanoma, with greater response numbers and less toxicity than IPI. PD-1 is a protein on the surface of activated T cells that triggers programmed cell death. If another molecule called PD-L1 binds to PD-1, the T cell dies or becomes docile. This is a way that the body regulates the immune system to avoid an overreaction. Many cancer cells make PD-L1 and can disarm the T cells, inhibiting them from attacking the tumor. Reported response rates show that medicines that block PD-1 or its partner molecule PD-L1 have a 30–40 percent response rate for melanoma patients. Unfortunately, not all patients respond to the PD-1 blockade, and work is underway to determine what specifically makes a person have a positive response.

The safety profile for the PD-1 blockade is remarkable, with milder toxicity associated with the treatment than Yervoy. Side effects include fatigue, rash, diarrhea, decreased appetite, nausea, and fever. The most worrying lethal side effect has been inflammation of the lungs (pneumonitis), and this is carefully

watched for and mitigated when possible. The therapy is given intravenously every two to three weeks. The FDA-approved Keytruda by Merck, a form of the PD-1 blockade, in September 2014. A product manufactured by Bristol-Myers Squibb, Nivolumab, marketed as Opdivo, was approved in December 2014 with the same restrictions as a third line therapy (you must have progressed on the other approved therapies) as Keytruda. Both should move to first line therapy early in 2015. To improve the response rate, clinical trials using combination strategies of the immunotherapy agents are underway. Mixing ipilimumab with the PD-1 blockade and/or with *BRAF*-inhibiting agents is showing some promising results in sequential trials, where each is given separately in different order.

The sky is the limit on how these immunotherapies and other agents may pan out, either alone, together, or sequentially. They have brought great optimism to a therapy that might keep melanoma under control for a durable response much like the combination of drugs has done for remission in AIDS.

TIL Therapy

TIL therapy, also known as ACT, adoptive cell transfer, is a therapy that uses tumor-infiltrating lymphocytes (TILs), and is of interest to many patients because of some reported full remissions. There are small trials ongoing at the National Cancer Institute and a few other cancer centers. The patients in these trials—most of whom have metastatic disease—usually have exhausted other treatment options, although some try it out the first time around in the course of their disease.

TIL therapy involves removing some of a patient's own immune-system cells, growing them in the laboratory, and infusing the cultured cells back into the patient's body. The idea is to provide an invading force of immune cells that can attack tumors in a way that the immune system has been incapable of doing on its own. The patient must first undergo chemotherapy to deplete the body of the current immune function and then get high-dose IL-2 with the infusion of T cells. This type of therapy requires hospitalization, as it can be risky and highly toxic. According to Dr. Keith Flaherty, MIF Scientific Advisory Board cochair, "The balance of efficacy and safety has not been established to consider the TIL therapy as an option in relation to immunotherapies and *BRAF* inhibitor-based therapy. Clinical trials, randomized to other therapies, are certainly lacking. It has been unclear whether the TIL therapy will be brought forward for consideration by regulatory agencies." Note: Dr. Flaherty, director of targeted therapies at Massachusetts General Hospital, made this comment in correspondence with the author.

Run by the National Cancer Institute, the National Institutes of Health's cost for the TIL therapy is said to be very high per patient. Funding is taxpayer underwritten. The high cost is due to lack of restrictions on the amount of scans and other procedures normally regulated by health insurance companies, as well as the labor-intensive therapy itself requiring many days of hospitalization. Several new biotech companies are forming around the concept of developing TIL therapy as a treatment approach and financing clinical trials, which could lead to approval. There is still a long way to go for this therapy, and the type of robust data needed to judge its merits may come in the near future. Other institutions (e.g., the Moffitt and MD Anderson cancer centers) have ACT programs, but have had difficulty replicating the response rate of the NCI. A major issue is that at the NIH, patients are very carefully selected to receive TIL treatment based on certain characteristics such as being young and fit, and that makes it difficult to be certain that the therapy would be effective for the majority of melanoma patients.

What Is the Abscopal Effect?

There is speculation, but only scant clinical data, that combining the immunotherapies (Yervoy and PD-1) with radiation treatment brings about a better response in distant metastasis. The *abscopal effect* is a phenomenon documented in patients in whom local radiation of a tumor is associated with the regression of metastatic cancer at a distance from the irradiated site. Until there is a greater amount of data from ongoing studies, we will not know whether this effect can result in improved response in the larger population of patients. In the meantime, many oncologists will treat a patient simultaneously with systemic immunotherapy and radiation in the hope that this expanded response will occur.

Clinical Trials

Clinical trials are an important option for treatment. Unfortunately, only about 3 percent of adult cancer patients enroll in trials. This may be due to fear of the unknown, or perhaps because the patient's doctor is not supportive of the idea. In fact, your oncologist should assist you in finding a trial at her location or elsewhere if you so desire. They are available at many cancer centers across the country and the world.

It can be a daunting task to discern which trials you qualify for and might be best for you. Some organizations may assist with this process, such as the National Cancer Institute and Melanoma International Foundation. Some general criteria that determine if you are likely to be eligible for any given trial include the following: (1) you are generally required to be eighteen years or older; (2) in general, you can't be too sick when you enter the trial—that is, you must be mobile; (3) patients with metastases in certain locations—the brain, for instance—may be disqualified; and (4) you may be required to not have had such previous treatment as chemotherapy or vaccines, or alternately a certain amount of time must have elapsed (a washout period) since your last treatment.

Inclusion and exclusion criteria may be confusing, and you should discuss the trial of interest closely with the research nurse. Unfortunately for patients, clinical trial design has not been updated in over fifty years. Hopefully, we will see more humane trial setups in the near future, including the restriction of:

- placebos (these are only effective for testing psychological drugs)
- ineffective drug comparison (e.g., using dacarbazine and other drugs we know have little response), trials that lack crossover to effective agents, or blinding of the agents used

Choosing to participate in a clinical trial can be a very difficult decision, especially if you have to face a randomized trial where you may be put into a group of patients who will receive a placebo or ineffective agent. Randomized trials can be a burdensome way to improve therapy. The best trials give us good therapy and help us improve it for others soon to be in our shoes.

Questions to Ask before Joining a Clinical Trial

When you contact the clinical trial coordinator, it is best to be prepared with good questions.

1. *What is the purpose of this study?*
2. *What phase is the study working in?* **Phase 1** usually tests toxicity and uses ever-increasing doses of the agent to find an acceptable one. **Phase 2** goes beyond the phase-one toxicity testing and looks for effectiveness of the drug in a particular cancer or group of cancers. **Phase 3** compares the new agent against standard treatment.
3. *What do previous studies of this therapy show?*
4. *Who is sponsoring the trial? How is it reviewed for safety?*

5. *What kinds of tests and treatments will we receive in the trial?*

6. *What are the potential side effects of the experimental treatment?* Get details about how the drug is administered and any results that relevant studies to date have shown about side effects.

7. *Is this a randomized trial?* This means participants are assigned by chance to separate groups that compare different treatments. Neither the participant nor the researcher can choose which group people are assigned to.

8. *Will some participants receive a placebo and others get the tested agent? If not, what other therapies are being given to compare efficacy? Is there crossover to the more effective agent should I progress?*

9. *Is the trial "double-blind," meaning that neither the doctor nor the patient knows what drug the patient is being given?*

10. *How will I pay for this? Will my insurance or the pharmaceutical company cover it?*

11. *How about travel and lodging expenses? How many days will I need to be at the office or hospital?*

12. *What happens once the trial is over? Will I continue on the medication? Will there be follow-up by the staff? Will I be told the results of the study?*

Your surgical or medical oncologist should be of great help in getting you to the point that you can make a decision about what to do—what option to choose, within or outside of the trial. The MIF provides patient navigation to help you choose a trial. You should know that you can leave the trial at any time. Also, if it is clear that you are getting worse, you may be given a different agent or be taken out of the trial.

What about Alternative Medicine?

One of the most dangerous practices among patients is not to disclose to their doctor any alternative or complementary medicines they have been taking. This risks interactions that could be serious. Just because a product says it is "all natural" doesn't mean it isn't a potent agent. An article published by Stephen Smith in the Boston Globe dated December 3, 2002, detailed the results from a Harvard University research group that spent three years reviewing more than four hundred published studies of therapies ranging from acupuncture, to megavitamins, to shark cartilage, to macrobiotic diets (http://rootandbranchom.com/References/References-CANCER-STUDY-OFFERS-GUIDE-TO-ALTERNATIVE-TREATMENTS.pdf). The goal of the study was to consider the impact of alternative treatments on both disease progression and survival, as well as on relief from the cancer or its treatment side effects. Only the treatment modality of mind-body therapy, such as relaxation training, meditation, yoga, and support groups, was found to be beneficial to cancer patients. Seven treatments, including moderate exercise, soy supplementation for prostate cancer, and acupuncture for chemotherapy-related nausea and vomiting, were given a qualified endorsement. It was determined that nine other treatments, including high-dose vitamins A and C, and St. John's wort, should be avoided by some cancer patients on the basis of being dangerous and possibly interacting negatively with chemotherapy and radiation.[7]

The message to take away from this study is that you shouldn't buy into those faraway treatments that claim a cure as long as you have a lot of money! Some cancer patients have been lured out or across the country with the promise of a cure for a price of $20,000 or more. Just remember that if it seems to be too good to be true, it probably is. Unfortunately, there are charlatans who are always quite willing to take advantage of patients in a desperate situation.

When There Are No Further Treatment Options Offered

Hope for controlling a life-threatening disease can be a devastating thing to give up when you are fighting an uncertain battle. However, many times doctors reach the end of their treatment modalities, and the patient may be so exhausted from going through treatment and having the disease continually recur that he may just want to take a break. Remember, the patient always has the right to say, "I've had enough."

No one can predict when someone might die, but usually there are indications that the treatment is not working and that palliative care, care that provides comfort thereby eliminating physical or spiritual pain, is the best course of action. The doctor may advise calling for hospice service and will place the orders for the service to start. Hospice is a remarkable concept designed to fulfill the hope for a pain-free dying experience without active interventions. It is made up of nurses and volunteers who visit the patient's home (there are also inpatient hospice services) to ensure that her pain is under control and she is comfortable. Usually, for hospice to take place, the doctor needs to certify that patient's death is likely within six months. However, to have hospice come in doesn't necessarily have to trigger funeral plans, although planning for a patient's funeral should be done when she's healthy and her mind is clear. Sometimes, end-stage patients learn of a clinical trial that they qualify for and become embroiled in health-insurance regulations that require them to choose between the active treatment and continuing hospice care. I would strongly argue that patients should be entitled to both simultaneously, especially when a hopeful clinical trial is embarked upon and there is still another chance for treatment. The problem is we have a system that focuses on either active therapy or palliative/hospice care and doesn't allow an appropriate interface between them. Additional flexibility would allow for patients to receive benefits from the palliative aspects of hospice care. Simultaneous care allowing a patient to undergo active treatment and have formal palliative care at the same time is ongoing in many cancer centers, such as the University of California at Davis Cancer Center. Hopefully, this will become a model for other centers and create a new trend in the future

Hospice home care, although wonderful, is often limited to a few nursing visits a week, and the rest of the care is limited to a volunteer visiting depending on the service you sign up for. Caregiving is exhausting and nearly 85 percent of families go it alone. Insurance doesn't cover nursing care beyond the limits of hospice care. This affects the special needs of cancer patients, such as not sleeping at night. A private-duty nurse to cover a night shift is prohibitively expensive for most families and is not covered by most insurance. One family I know took shifts to provide around-the-clock care for their dad, who had many restless nights before he died. They were fortunate to have many able-bodied, caring people to carry out this task, whereas in another family only the husband was willing and able to help out. He left his job to be an around-the-clock nurse for three months until his wife died. He later suffered from post-traumatic stress disorder and needed extensive psychological counseling and time to recuperate.

A Caregiver's Prescription

If you find yourself as the primary caregiver, try to follow these guidelines from *Improving Palliative Care for Cancer*,[8] so that you don't deplete yourself.

1. Choose to take charge of your life and don't let your loved one's illness always take center stage.
2. Remember to be good to yourself. Love, honor, and value yourself. You're doing a very hard job and deserve some quality time just for you.
3. Watch for signs of depression in yourself and don't delay in getting professional help when you need it.
4. When people offer to help, accept the offer and suggest specific things that they can do. Develop a plan of care and assign specific tasks to family members.

5. Educate yourself about your loved one's condition, as this information can empower you and enable you to work more effectively with professionals.

6. There's a difference between caring and doing. Be open to technologies and ideas that promote your loved one's independence.

7. Trust your instincts. Most of the time they'll lead you in the right direction.

8. Grieve for your losses and then allow yourself to dream new dreams.

9. Stand up for your rights as a caregiver.

10. Seek support from other caregivers. You can gather strength from knowing you are not alone.

One final note: a person should have the opportunity to die at home if he or she expresses that desire and it is not a burden to maintain quality care there. The dying person doesn't necessarily need to be isolated in a sick room, either. One of my dear friends, John, had melanoma, and it was a quick progression from a recurrence in the form of brain metastases to his death. His death, although unhappily met, was still a beautiful thing. John's wife called me to say she thought he was close to dying and asked whether I might want to say good-bye. Besides being friends since our kids were in school together, I had helped in their journey from when the mole was first spotted on his neck to the day the oncologist suggested hospice. I stopped by to visit, and my first thought was, "Where's John?" The room was full of people chatting and mingling, and then I spotted him. He was sitting on the couch in the living room in the midst of the crowd. Many friends and family were sitting close, holding his hand, and talking to him. He was free of pain, assisted by oxygen to breathe easier. After I left, I thought long and hard about John, considering whether this should be the way death occurs. I had encountered only one other death at home, and the person was isolated coldly to a distant room. I decided that John's family had found a healthy way to handle a very sad, yet natural, occurrence in life, and I believe it will have a lasting impression on their four children, possibly making their grieving process just a little bit easier down the road.

CHAPTER 6

The Patient Experience: The Stories

Cancer is feared more than death in our society. Melanoma seems especially ominous to some, but is lightly dismissed as "just skin cancer" by others. In reality, melanoma is menacing because no sure or easy treatment exists once it has spread beyond the initial site.

To put the potential outcomes in perspective, it might be helpful to understand the actual impact on lives by sharing the journeys of real melanoma patients. The first story is my own and shows how I contended with a stage II melanoma during pregnancy. The second story is that of Shirley Zaremba, who was diagnosed with stage III C melanoma. Following Shirley's story are stories of stage IV patients who each had different therapies, yet are all living active, happy lives with little or no disease. Prior to 2012, stage IV disease was considered the end of the road. You will find the stories here to be quite to the contrary. (To see some of these patients tell their stories, download our video "Never Walk This Path Alone" on the Melanoma International Foundation (MIF) website at http://melanomainternational.org/events-webinar/patient-experience-video

www.melanomainternational.org or e-mail the MIF, at contact@melanomainternational.org for a USB drive of the video.)

My Story

The 1988 holiday season was fading, and so was I. I was five months pregnant and suffering from the flu. Because I was a busy freelance writer with an active toddler, it was a rare occasion for me to stretch out on the couch in my nightgown as I did that afternoon. For some reason, while lying on my side I glanced at the back of my leg. To my surprise, a band of little black bubbles appeared to be growing out of what I had always thought was a birthmark. Instinctively I knew this was something to be concerned about. The warning signs of cancer were familiar to me. This was definitely an "obvious change in a mole."

The next morning, I went to a dermatologist. We were both pregnant, our bellies nearly brushing in the small examination room, and she had no room to hide her alarmed reaction to the suspicious growth on my leg. She called a surgeon to get me in for a biopsy. After injecting a local anesthetic, the surgeon cut out the mole, along with some tissue underneath and around it, and closed the wound with a few stitches. The procedure was quick and painless.

Waiting for the answer from the hospital pathology department was torture. I felt that my existence hinged on the results. As the days wore on, I couldn't eat or sleep. I was anxious about losing my pregnancy or, worse, dying after I gave birth, abandoning my newborn and two-year-old.

After two weeks of living in suspense, I finally called and urged the surgeon to send the biopsy to a teaching hospital in Philadelphia for a faster response. In less than twenty-four hours, Wallace Clark, MD, a pathologist at the University of Pennsylvania, determined that it was melanoma. (Dr. Clark, who passed away in 1997, was a brilliant melanoma pathologist.)

When the dermatologist called me with the news, I felt disembodied as she sympathetically advised surgery and suggested that I see a specialist in Philadelphia. I then called my family doctor, also a friend, for a list of surgeons. His voice faltered, making him sound more upset about the diagnosis than I was (which was totally out of character for him). The reactions of both doctors really sent me into a panic. Next I called my nurse-midwife. She sounded worried, too. But she provided reassurance when she read to me from one of her nursing texts about melanoma. The book said that women often have a better prognosis than men, especially with a melanoma located on a lower extremity. That tiny piece of information would keep my spirits up for a long time. That was 1989, but little has changed for this to be a positive prognostic indicator.

I needed more information, though—the Internet was yet to be—and I obtained it from the National Cancer Institute's Cancer Information Service hotline. The hotline supplied a list of melanoma specialists in the Philadelphia area. Note: this hotline currently only refers patients to the Melanoma International Foundation as a resource. I had a choice of two doctors: DuPont Guerry or the one my dermatologist had mentioned, and that's where I ended up.

I still wasn't sure about my prognosis and didn't know exactly what treatment I needed. As my husband waited with me to see the doctor, I noticed him looking very worried for the first time as he checked out the chemo lounge chairs in the waiting area. I couldn't help but feel that at last he was validating my anxiety.

My husband was allowed into the examination room with me. I wanted him there to help remember the details. Although I felt on top of things with my list of prepared questions, my mind seemed shrouded in a fog. Sometimes I would ask a question and not even listen to the answer.

I liked the doctor—he was kind, and willing to discuss everything in great detail. I was relieved when he suggested a further surgery that could be performed at our local hospital: a simple procedure of taking off additional skin around the site of the melanoma to ensure that all the malignant cells had been removed. From the pathology report, he surmised that I had an 80 percent chance of surviving eight years, whereas Dr. Clark's estimate on my pathology report had been 90 percent. I liked Dr. Clark's odds better, but I really wanted a 100 percent chance!

The next hurdle was to find a surgeon quickly, since the doctors were acting as if there was some urgency. The surgeon I chose was bright, young, and flexible about my terms: local anesthesia, no extended hospital stay, and no drugs that might compromise my pregnancy. This surgeon was very cheerful about my prognosis, saying, "These things rarely ever come back." The next week I went into the hospital for surgery. The surgeon was late, and I waited way beyond the usual twenty-four hours of fasting for the procedure. Being pregnant and having only a local anesthetic, I begged for some ice chips and was granted this eventually.

In the operating room, I was quite awake and actually had a choice in the music for the procedure. I though the classical choice would be most relaxing. The surgeon took off a two-centimeter (three-quarter-inch) strip of skin around the biopsy scar—more than needed to be removed. (Had I read this book first, it would have been half that.) I had to have a skin graft from my hip to close the wound. A nurse held my hand during the procedure and shared with me that one of the doctors on staff had recently died of melanoma. And if that wasn't bad enough, the procedure sounded like a chainsaw vibrating through my whole body, as a piece of my skin was being shimmed off and grafted onto my leg.

My recuperation was steady, and the deadline I had to meet for a magazine cover story kept me sane. The pain from the skin graft was the worst part, and I totally avoided the use of painkillers because of my pregnancy. I did take a shot of brandy on the worst night of pain. I also found it difficult, in my third trimester, to adjust to walking on crutches. A few months later, I returned to the teaching hospital for a follow-up examination. This visit was upsetting because I wasn't able to see the same doctor—even after requesting him in advance—and because no family members were permitted in the examination room. The final blow came when this doctor told me that I should not plan to breastfeed my baby. I called the Pigmented Lesion Clinic at the University of Pennsylvania and was assured that breastfeeding would not make my disease reappear, as the other doctor had insinuated.

At almost nine months pregnant in sweltering June weather, I didn't feel like going anywhere too far from home. I had gained forty pounds and couldn't even bend over to plug in a fan. But we made the trip to Philadelphia to meet DuPont Guerry, one of the doctors recommended by the NCI at the University of Pennsylvania.

At that time, the clinic was housed in a drab old building with stained linoleum hallways. The elevator was not to be trusted. Despite the tacky appearance of the place, we were greeted by a warm, family-oriented staff who welcomed my husband and daughter into the examination room.

Dr. Guerry, director PENNs melanoma program, talked so fast that he nearly erased his slight Southern drawl. But despite his rush to get to his next patient, he was willing to answer all my questions. His prognosis was confusing and filled with statistics, but he reassured me in a very clear manner that I was likelier to get killed on the Schuylkill Expressway than by melanoma. In taking my history, Dr. Guerry asked if I had had many sunburns as a child. I recounted growing up in Arizona and having my mother, on several occasions, soothe my sun-scorched skin by dabbing it with cotton soaked in iced tea. I also remembered dreading our family vacations at the beach. I always had to stay fully clothed because otherwise I would burn badly, even when I was up to my neck in the ocean.

The doctor explained that if the unlikely happened and the melanoma in my system spread, it would probably go to the lymph nodes in my groin area, most likely within the next two to three years. I was to return in three months to get a chest X-ray after my baby was born.

A few weeks later, I gave birth to a beautiful ten-pound baby boy, apparently unscathed by my tangle with melanoma. The surgeon had issued a directive to my midwife to have the placenta sectioned by the pathology department at the local hospital. As he explained, the pathology needed to be performed because melanoma is one of the few cancers that can cross the placenta and affect the fetus. Since Dr. Guerry assured me that this result had been reported only in cases where the mother had widespread melanoma, I declined to have this step performed.

I returned to Dr. Guerry a few months later for an extensive workup. It was slightly humiliating to have the clinic's photographer take pictures of my naked postpartum body from head to toe, getting a close-up of my funny-looking mole. The doctor explained that the photos would be used for comparison with photos taken on subsequent visits so that the physicians could look for changes that might herald a second melanoma.

At one of my checkups, still just a few years since diagnosis, Dr. Guerry said, after examining me, "Now get out of here, because you're too damned healthy to be here." That meant a lot to me; I knew the potentially dire consequences of a recurrence. I've been fortunate to remain healthy and melanoma-free for the past twenty-five years. (Dr. Guerry is now retired and couldn't be convinced to do a third book with me)

Shirley Zaremba and I first met when she and her husband called the Melanoma International Foundation's helpline to ask about her stage III diagnosis and the therapy that was recommended. We soon became good friends. Shirley had a mole on her left big toe that had been present since birth. When she dropped a box on the toe at work, the mole started to bleed and did not heal, so she decided to get it checked out. The day before her appointment with a dermatologist, she felt a lump in her groin. A fine needle aspiration confirmed the lymph node to contain melanoma cells. The diagnosis was acral melanoma, more than ten millimeters deep. Her toe was amputated and a full node dissection was completed on her groin, where there was a matted cluster of nodes. The doctors pushed hard to start a course of interferon after the surgical wound healed.

Shirley recounts her perspective on the melanoma at that point: "I felt the surgery had removed it and I was a strong believer in keeping my immune system healthy and avoiding harsh treatments." At the three-year mark, Shirley had a recurrence of a melanoma tumor on her shin, and the tumor was surgically removed. She is now eight years out from the original surgery and five years from the recurrence. According to Shirley, "I am doing great, except for the lymphedema [a chronic swelling and fluid retention from the lymph node dissection that prevents her from returning to work]." Shirley says, "I continue to appreciate the things I once took for granted and [I am] now a grandmother six times over, loving every minute of it." Shirley also comes to the MIF forum frequently to reassure and educate other stage III patients.

Richard Kaminski

Richard is a survivor of four different cancers, including melanoma. He and his wife have been married for forty-three years and feel blessed to have a daughter, son, daughter-in-law, and grandbaby. During an eye exam in 1998, the doctor spotted an unusual mole on Richard's face and recommended he see a dermatologist. The mole was removed, and he started a regimen of annual X-rays and checkups.

Eleven years later, a persistent cough led Richard to get a CAT scan, two needle biopsies, and a PET scan. He was diagnosed with stage IV melanoma and underwent a grueling treatment of IL-2 (interleukin 2) therapy. When his cancer was found to be advancing still, he found a clinical trial for the *B-rafF* inhibitor Zelboraf, which he started in March of 2010. The B-raf protein is a key component of the cellular pathways and may become mutated and cause tumor growth. New BRAFtherapies target this mutation to eliminate tumor progression.

During the experimental treatment, (the now-approved *BRAF*therapy Zelboraf) his tumors continued to shrink in size to about 4 percent of their original size and have remained that way for four years to this day in 2015. Richard currently continues on the clinical trial and lives an active, happy life. In 2014, he was found to have an early melanoma that was removed with wide excision and dismissed as resolved.

Richard explains the importance of having a support network when dealing with disease: "When fighting melanoma, you need a support team to help you day to day, month to month, and hopefully, year to year. For me, the support team comes in the form of a pyramid. At the top is my wife providing me with continuous support and energy and we have family and friends to share with. I'm also fortunate to be in the care of a great medical team. A little further down the pyramid are other melanoma patients participating in clinical trials; there is a good feeling that information you are providing will be able to help others. Online support groups provide a base of firsthand knowledge and support such as the MIF forum. And lastly, the researchers and support people who work tirelessly to find new treatments."

Alicia Tagliaferro

Alicia was first diagnosed with melanoma in 1990, a few months after her son was born. She had surgery to remove the mole and moved on with her life. Three years later, melanoma was found in a lymph node, and several nodes were removed. She enrolled in a clinical trial for interferon but was placed in the placebo group. So Alicia took a more aggressive approach and opted for the dacarbazine, or DTIC, but stopped at the third cycle.

In 1998, Alicia had been disease-free for five years when she became pregnant. Her daughter was born in 1999, and according to Alicia, "Life was good!" Four years later, a damper was put on Alicia's life when she found out that the melanoma had metastasized to her left lung. Enrolling in a clinical trial, she again was randomized to the placebo arm. Four months later, lower back pain sent Alicia for a CAT scan, and a tumor was found on her lumbar spine. The tumor was removed by radiation and surgery, but follow-up scans showed a small tumor in her brain. The tumor and an additional brain lesion were successfully treated with stereotactic radiation. To add to the burden Alicia faced, melanoma invaded her small bowel, twice requiring surgery. With little choice of treatments available, the option of the pharmaceutical Leukine, a synthetic version of a granulocyte macrophage colony-stimulating factor (GM-CSF), was presented. According to Alicia, "This was a very difficult time, as I knew too well that treatment options were limited for central nervous system disease and most clinical trials excluded patients with this history." Patients with brain or central nervous system disease are often excluded from clinical trials because of poor prognosis. This has changed with the advent of successful brain radiation techniques, such as CyberKnife and Gamma Knife. A webinar on this subject by Yale neurosurgeon Veronica Chiang is presented on the website of Melanoma International Foundation at http://melanomainternational.org/webinar/2012/01/radiation-treatment-in-brain-metastases.

Alicia started GM-CSF in 2005 and continued her self-injections for two years. "My doctors and I believe this therapy was the kick my immune system needed to keep the disease at bay." And, happily, it has, with Alicia showing no evidence of disease ten years later. "I developed a partnership with my doctors and that was instrumental in achieving the best outcome. Being a long-term survivor is a blessing and I am very grateful for every new day that I am alive. I was able to have a daughter, see my son graduate from high school and college, and I hope my story can bring hope to everyone who is diagnosed with melanoma."

Jamie Troil Goldfarb

Jamie's primary melanoma was found on her left thigh in January 2007. It was removed, and the sentinel-node biopsy confirmed no further evidence of disease in the nodes. However, over the next year, she had three infections near the site of her surgery that the surgeon assured her were not related to melanoma. After her continued persistence, Jamie's oncologist insisted she revisit the surgeon, who agreed to reexcise the area. This biopsy was conclusive that there was a recurrence of the melanoma. After receiving clear scans and consulting with specialists and her oncologist, Jamie was advised that no further treatment was necessary but that she would continue to be closely observed. That was in 2009, and Jamie became pregnant, giving birth to a healthy boy.

A year after the all-clear signal in December 2009, Jamie was diagnosed with melanoma in her liver and pancreas. She entered a clinical trial at the National Institutes of Health for TIL therapy, or Adoptive Cell Therapy, using tumor-infiltrating lymphocytes. While waiting for the trial to start, she underwent treatment with the standard of care, dacarbazine, or DTIC.

But between April and August of 2011, even though she was receiving the preliminary treatment, Jamie developed thirty-five additional subcutaneous tumors. She started on the TIL therapy in September 2012 and was declared disease-free in September 2014. Jamie offers this advice: "You can't rest until you have researched all of your treatment options and speak to specialists before you make a decision. The good news is melanoma research is changing so rapidly; what a wonderful thing that is!" Jamie kept a wonderful account of her journey in an online blog, www.melanoma-mom.com with her Thanksgiving 2014 post reporting she is still cancer-free.

T. J. Sharpe

T. J. was first diagnosed with multiple tumors in many organs in 2012. Tests confirmed the presence of tumors in his lungs, spleen, liver, and an eight-centimeter one pressing against his small bowel. Stage IV melanoma was the diagnosis. T. J. lost thirty pounds, had the tumor on his small bowel removed, and started preparing for a long battle with cancer. Testing confirmed that this was a recurrence of a malignant melanoma that had been removed twelve years prior, in 2000. He started a blog called *Patient #1*, so named because he was the first patient to enter a TIL trial using the newly approved drugs Yervoy and IL-2.

The TIL trial allowed him to recover temporarily, but the disease recurred a few months later. The seventh dose of IL-2 was his last; the doctors detected the beginnings of lung failure, heart failure, and liver dysfunction. He came to the MIF to help him with navigation. Searching for plan B options for drugs helped him find a trial for the PD-1 therapy— a therapy that blocks the natural immunologic response of programmed cell death—right in his Florida neighborhood. Luckily, he was randomized in the trial to the PD-1 drug instead of the chemotherapy arm of the trial. He has been cautiously optimistic, as this trial produced a 60 percent tumor shrinkage during the course of the year. He did have a recurrence in the form of a tumor growing on his adrenal gland, but the tumor was surgically removed, and he was able to continue the PD-1 blockade infusions after the surgery. On his blog, T. J. shares the "optimistic prism of a patient who is on the long and winding road towards overcoming melanoma's long odds and potentially deadly consequences." In his spare time, he continues to enjoy his active family life with two little ones and his wife.

Jonathan Friedlaender

Jonathan first discovered his melanoma in 1996. He had a wide excision and sentinel-node biopsy that showed negative nodes for melanoma. But despite the findings he continued to have positive nodes removed until a complete node dissection in 2008. In 2009, Jonathan got the news that he was stage IV. He was put on interferon and IL-2, but had no response to either therapy.

In 2010, he started receiving IPI (ipilimumab) and responded for eighteen months. During this time, three small brain metastases cropped up, but they were zapped with stereotactic radiation (SRS). In 2012, he entered the CureTech 011 PD-1 blockade trial and had no response. Then he went back to IPI for a second round but continued to have no response. A third round of IPI was prescribed combined with Sylatron (a type of interferon) and still he had no response. He enrolled in a trial using the ADC (DEDN6526A) therapy, a chemo-targeted therapy that is still in the pipeline but may be discontinued. That was a phase 1 trial, and he responded for ten months. Another small brain metastasis was then detected, and again, SRS was used.

Jonathan started the PD-1 blockade drug Keytruda in May of 2014 in an expanded-access program and was responsive three months later. He underwent extensive abdominal surgery and was hospitalized for more than two months. But since continuing on Keytruda after recovering from a rough summer, he has had a happier fall with no progression of disease.

According to Jonathan, "So, all in all, I am feeling as though I've likely weathered the worst and am beginning to experience the pleasures of life again, although a couple of months ago I really was looking over the abyss and in a lot of pain. I had a great seventy-fourth birthday last weekend with my two grown kids and granddaughter, and an old buddy of mine is talking about possible new research collaborations in the coming years—unthinkable discussions a few months ago. Life can be fun again, and I have a wonderful wife to enjoy it with."

Stephen Connor

Stephen was first diagnosed when a tiny speck on his neck was determined to be positive for melanoma. He had a sentinel-node biopsy, which came out negative for melanoma. Two years later, a scan showed spots on his lung, but they were too small to remove. He was given IL-2, and after two separate rounds, the melanoma lesions did not respond. Seven brain lesions were identified and Stephen proceeded with Gamma Knife treatment in August of 2013. In September he began IPI treatment, and after four sessions it was found that he had three new brain lesions. After receiving Gamma Knife treatment again, he had clean scans from January 2014 until May 2014. But in June, a new brain lesion showed up. He entered a clinical trial using a PD-1 blockade for patients with brain metastases. As of August 2014, his scans showed a 60 percent reduction in lung lesions, and the brain lesion is stable. An MRI from October 2014 showed that the brain lesion had shrunk by 60 percent. Stephen, like Jonathan, had a long and rough journey.

His perspective is this: "Although this period has been difficult for me and my family, there have been some benefits. I've had a chance to strengthen relationships with family and friends; I have reconnected with old friends and have made new friends. I am a very open, nonprivate person and don't keep many secrets. When people, sometimes even those I don't know, ask how I'm doing, I'll usually let them know about my illness. I do have reservations about overwhelming people with my problems, but I find this approach cathartic and it helps me to better accept and manage my situation."

The above patients demonstrate the importance of becoming an empowered patient. We work hard to educate patients about options and to understand their disease. You can put a face to these stories on the MIF Video, Never Walk This Path Alone available free of charge by writing to contact@melanomainternational.org. It is available in a small USB drive.

CHAPTER 7

Tending to Your Spirits

Courage is not the absence of fear, but the triumph over it.
—Nelson Mandela

*N*elson Mandela lived well into his nineties despite suffering a torturous life of twenty-seven years in prison, where he was well acquainted with facing fear. The rollercoaster ride of any serious illness instills much anxiety, but learning to triumph over it by gaining knowledge can smooth out the journey.

Half the battle against cancer is psychological. The waiting is the hardest part for a person dealing with melanoma or any other cancer. Over and over, normal life is put on hold because of the disease. First, the patient is in limbo until the initial biopsy results are made available. Then the phone call arrives with your diagnosis. Next comes the nervous waiting from scans to checkup to learn whether any recurrence has been detected. If the disease does make a comeback, the patient must wait again—this time for the results of the diagnostic tests. Then there is a decision to make about the next treatment usually after surgery and the biopsy results. Meanwhile, the mind works overtime as the patient imagines every conceivable outcome, from best to worst. To make matters still more difficult, family members and health care providers may overreact during this process or be unsure about the most desirable course of treatment. All these factors contribute to the patient feeling out of control and helpless in dealing with the situation. In the past, cancer patients were kept out of the loop, merely passive observers of their care, because the physician and family members kept the details of their treatment and life expectancy a closely guarded secret. Fortunately, the trend these days is for patients to be actively involved in their treatment. I highly recommend that you make a point of working in full partnership with your physician. Not only will you receive better care, you will take a step toward conquering your fear of the unknown by gathering knowledge and gaining some measure of control during a very vulnerable time in your life.

In coping with melanoma, you will probably manage your fear in whatever style you generally adopt in a crisis. You should proceed in the way that makes you feel most comfortable. I remember the hardest time for me (before I knew my prognosis) was when I first woke up in the morning. As I gained consciousness, the realization that I may be facing death would slowly set in and so would the tension in my mind and body. The resources and ideas I present in this chapter are intended to make you feel more at ease in dealing with your melanoma, no matter what your prognosis.

Peace of Mind

If you're lucky, the physician or melanoma clinic you visit may offer care for your psychological needs. University-based hospitals normally have psychological services available or can at least provide referrals to appropriate therapists. There are professional organizations as well. The APOS (American Psychological Oncology Society) has a toll-free helpline: 1-866-276-7443 (1-866-APOS-4-HELP). This line is a national resource to help cancer patients and their caregivers find emotional support in their own communities.

If your clinic or doctor doesn't bring up psychological care as a part of your treatment and you feel the need, request a recommendation for a therapist who counsels cancer patients. Good physicians can usually sense distress in patients by asking a question or two, and figure out which ones need their spirits attended to. If the patient wants to discuss unresolved issues with a therapist or if during the examination the physician detects a need for counseling, the patient should be referred to a specialist. Insurance rarely covers this, or pays for only a small portion, which is very unfortunate. We can only hope that one day there will be more acceptance of the importance of the mind/body connection to wellness.

Dr. Arlene Houldin, RN, PhD, is an experienced psychosocial oncology consultant who previously headed the oncology nursing program at the University of Pennsylvania and currently runs a nonprofit home-health agency (www.healconsulting.org). This is how she describes her work with patients:

> I support people through a tough time—basically by providing supportive therapy, teaching coping techniques, decision-making, and problem-solving skills—and assist in resolving family issues. There's frequently a sublevel of anger and blame that needs to be dealt with, sometimes involving blame for sun-worshipping habits, much like the guilt associated with smoking and lung cancer. Melanoma is horribly disruptive, because it often hits younger people who are just raising their families, heavily into career goals, with lots of financial burdens. And sometimes they are even caring for older family members, and suddenly they're struck down by this illness, disrupting their own personal plans and the family in a major way. So melanoma can involve a lot more family issues to deal with than some other cancers.

Dr. Houldin points out that "this is not the time to confront patients with ways to cope that are foreign to them, because if you do, you will lose their trust." (Quotes taken from personal interviews with Dr. Houldin.)

But if you stick your head in the ground and don't get proper medical follow-up, that may cause you to miss the opportunity of finding something you can do that will help you—like researching new therapies or joining a clinical trial. With denial of the disease, you may miss the opportunity for emotional stability or spiritual growth that comes from working through whatever happens with loved ones, friends, and counselors and physicians. I know from my own experience that my body and mind were experiencing the "fight or flight" response, where you act reactively more than cognitively. One case in particular that taught me patiencewas a pediatrician who knew just enough about melanoma to scare herself about a bruised thumbnail. She was certain it was acral lentiginous melanoma, as she didn't remember injuring herself. I spoke with her sometimes two or three times a day on the MIF helpline until the problem resolved, reassuring her that it was highly unlikely to be this type of melanoma, but helping her get to a specialist who could tell for sure. I never discount what a patient might feel is wrong since you just don't know anything for certain with the human body.

Jon Kabat-Zinn, PhD, professor of medicine emeritus at the University of Massachusetts Medical School, and creator of the Stress Reduction Clinic and the Center for Mindfulness in Medicine, Health Care, and Society, pioneered the mindful meditation approach to ease the stressed-out mind. His books and CDs are widely available, as are programs that teach mindful meditation. His theory is based on clearing your mind of distractions and avoiding focusing on the past or future. He suggests that living "in the moment" can help quell the anxiety of disease possibilities. Mindfulness practice helps break that cycle of ruminating thinking, where you overthink your situation and wear yourself down.

Strength in Numbers

Not all people are cut out for support groups. Many find it hard to open up to a group of people they hardly know. I found joining a support group a daunting undertaking after my initial diagnosis partly because I was afraid someone in the group would die. That being said, support groups do often provide a safe environment where, as one participant put it, "You can't scare each other." A good many of the group members may already have weathered what you are going through, and will usually allow you to express whatever you want without reacting judgmentally; something friends and family may have trouble doing.

Some studies strongly suggest that people who participate in support groups live longer than those who don't. One of the most compelling studies is by psychiatrist David Spiegel of Stanford University.[1] In trying to disprove that psychological factors affect cancer, he compared the vital statistics of participants in his breast cancer support groups with those of other nonparticipants. He found that the women in the support group survived eighteen months longer on average than those who didn't join a support group. He attributes the increased longevity primarily to what he calls the grandmother effect: people who feel cared for and are being taken care of by others often avoid harmful habits—they eat, sleep, and exercise well, thereby fortifying their body's ability to fight illness. He attributes a similar mechanism to explain why married men live longer than single men.

Spiegel also monitored immune function in an attempt to confirm the results of the first study and could not validate the results. What *is* known is that cancer patients, on average, suffer higher rates of depression and anxiety. If a person is isolated, they may have low morale and will be less likely to take good care of themselves. That's why it is important to build a support network of friends and family.

Studies on melanoma and the effect of psychological interventions have been published by F. I. Fawzy, professor of psychiatry at the University of California at Los Angeles. Fawzy and colleagues examined the outcome of sixty-eight melanoma patients who were participants in a six-week support group. They found that patients not in support groups had a higher death rate than those receiving psychological support from a group.[2] In 2003, Fawzy revisited this study, examining the survival benefits for the same sixty-eight patients with melanoma at the ten-year mark. Fawzy found the survival benefit of the structured psychiatric group intervention to have weakened, but not disappeared, by the tenth year. Being male and having a greater Breslow levelwere predictive of poorer outcome (something we know to be true from current melanoma mortality data). But after adjusting for these factors, there still remained a significant difference for those in the support group.

Despite this research claiming that support groups do not have a significant survival benefit, there is a considerable amount of evidence suggesting that support groups improve the quality of life for cancer patients. Better coping skills, improved self-esteem, less anxiety, and improved mood are noted benefits. These are highly valuable psychosocial attributes for a patient to take away from therapy. Quality of life, although measured less frequently by research than quantity of life, is equally or possibly more important for the cancer patient.

If you decide to join a support group, you may have trouble finding one specifically geared to melanoma. If you want to start your own melanoma support group, you usually can find a place to meet rent-free, such as in a public library conference room, a doctor's office, or hospital meeting room. Location is a very important consideration, since people undergoing therapy, in addition to all of the other time-consuming stressors in their lives, are not going to trek to a faraway spot. Having the group meet where melanoma patients receive therapy is one solution, but sometimes a more domestic location is preferred. You can switch locations monthly to meet the geographic reach of everyone in the group, but make sure you meet at least once a month on the same designated day. You can advertise the support group in oncology/dermatology offices, hospitals, newspapers, and on the radio and Internet. Equally important to finding a good location and people to join is the facilitator chosen to moderate the group. The biggest expense you will probably encounter will be the group facilitator's fee, but don't balk at that—smooth group functioning will depend on the guidance of someone with a solid counseling background. Each participant could chip in a nominal amount to cover the expense or perhaps you could find an oncology/dermatology practice, pharmaceutical provider, or corporate entity that will sponsor the group. You may also want to designate the support group in one setting as being open only to people at certain stages of disease—perhaps stages 1 and 2—and another group in a different setting as accepting people stages 3 and 4. This will probably increase the comfort level of participants.

Many swear by web-based support groups to get the support they need. This appears to be a growing trend. However, I am troubled by the misinformation about the disease and lack of professional oversight on these bulletin boards. Online support groups should be used with caution, as these venues cannot always assure privacy or confidentiality, and the group leaders may have no special training or qualifications, especially if the group takes place in an unmonitored chat room. You should look further into these issues before choosing a support group and make sure you choose a reputable organization that manages these issues carefully to protect participants. The MIF offers a moderated forum at http://www.melanomaforum.org where you can feel confident that the information provided is scientifically validated and your personal information will never be shared.

Family and Friends

How your family and friends react to your diagnosis may present unexpected problems. Families under stress communicate inefficiently or in bizarre ways. You may find loved ones responding with unaccustomed behavior—for example, denial and avoidance. However your family ordinarily functions, honest, open communication is ultimately the most comforting for all involved. All of us have a sixth sense about when people aren't being candid with us, and especially when those closest to us are being untruthful. Families make the mistake of hiding information, and in the communication dodging, either the person with the illness or the family members think things are worse than they are, and the whole family avoids talking about the issues. Family members are often hardest to communicate with because of long-established patterns of interaction. Sometimes the emotional ties may even be too strong. If you are having problems talking about your illness with your family, a therapist who specializes in crisis counseling can facilitate better communication.

The Mind-Body Connection

Another psychological trap, akin to the perceived need to paint a rosy portrait for your family, originates with the mistaken belief that people get cancer (or provoke a recurrence) by not coping right or by handling stress badly. This is a myth. You cannot get cancer—or aggravate it once you have it—by thinking particular thoughts. All the talk of mind over body makes patients feel guilty and responsible for their cancer in the belief that maybe they caused their disease by not coping with life the right way. Our society makes us feel that our survival is up to us. But there really isn't any proof of this. Scientific evidence that coping styles do not influence cancer outcomes echoes the theme of accepting rather than trying to change a patient's coping method. An article by Dr. M. Pettigrew published in the British Medical Journal, found after reviewing twenty-six studies on the effects of psychological coping styles on recurrence and survival that there is no correlation. Coping styles were defined as either fighting spirit or hopelessness/helplessness.3

Dr. Houldin points out that many patients, influenced by publications that stress positive thinking, are filled with guilt because they imagine that the inability to cope has brought on their cancer:

While those books can be enormously helpful, sometimes they carry a hidden message of guilt: "If I'm not positive all the time, my cancer will get worse or come back." Clearly, the scientific evidence doesn't show that. People should not be beating themselves up at this time of crisis. Unfortunately, some families will use this mind-body theory to keep patients under control, saying, "You're not being positive enough (or, you're not being cheerful enough), so you won't get better." Here people are, dealing with the diagnosis of the illness, the treatment, and the uncertainty of having it, and then they have to be positive all of the time. Cancer patients need to be given permission to be upset and grieve and vent their negative feelings.

Worrying about Your Body

In addition to allowing yourself to be upset, give yourself permission to be a hypochondriac or hypervigilant about your body, too. As if it isn't enough to deal with all the pressure to be happy and positive at this time of disease, you are also forced to tune in to your body more than ever before. Your confidence in your immune system is definitely going to be shaky; after all, if your body let you down once, it might do it again. Every little symptom may drive you crazy thinking about whether it is a recurrence or spread of melanoma. Doctors inexperienced in cancer treatment may not be sensitive to this issue and may dismiss your concerns or scare you needlessly. I remember initially thinking that swollen lymph nodes in my neck might be metastasized melanoma. My most recent scare, fifteen years out from my diagnosis, came in the form of a swollen lymph node in my groin. I have a wonderful general practitioner who palpated the node and was certain it was just a reaction to an infection/. I also called Dr. Guerry and he asked which side of my body it was on—because it was on the opposite side from where my melanoma had occurred, he confirmed there was no need to worry. Still, if you have a gut feeling that something *is* going on, don't worry about looking ridiculous. Talk about it with your doctor and get it checked so that you can stop worrying. And switch doctors if your queries are met with patronizing remarks or dismissed too easily. Take comfort in the idea that sooner or later your feelings about your body will normalize.

In the Long Run

When I was first diagnosed, I really needed to calm down. I was pregnant, so any medication was out of the question. What helped me was to practice yoga, meditation, deep breathing, and other relaxation techniques. I couldn't exercise after surgery because of the crutches, but as soon as I was healed I walked as often as possible. I believe all of these measures helped me cope better. Frequently, antidepressant or antianxiety medications are prescribed to help deal with the initial shock of being diagnosed with a life-threatening illness. I believe these drugs can be very useful, but aren't necessarily a magic bullet to cure anxiety and depression. Talk therapy should be considered an important treatment in conjunction with the medication.

You should also bear in mind that your doctor is a human being who doesn't have any magical powers to cure you, and certainly doesn't have all of the answers all of the time. Giving yourself permission to be upset will actually help regulate your emotional reactions. Cry and laugh often. It's OK to feel sorry for yourself and to feel scared. It will be especially beneficial if you can confront the issues that upset and frighten you and then process them emotionally. Don't be afraid to ask for help from either a professional therapist or those close to you. This is a lot to handle on your own.

Many cancer patients are ultimately thankful to be brought face to face with their own mortality because for the first time in their lives they get their priorities straight. The other challenges encountered in life may seem trivial by comparison. And despite how the initial quaking makes you feel, you will emerge from this ordeal on a stronger foundation than you ever imagined.

Glossary

acral lentiginous melanoma. A type of melanoma that appears among both whites and people of color. It is most often found in the thumb and big toe, but also appears on the soles of feet and palms of hands. It is called subungual when found in the nail bed. Late detection often results in a worse prognosis, as it is a rare type of melanoma not often seen by physicians.

actinic keratosis (AK). A small, scaly red patch caused by sun exposure; it is potential precancer of the nonmelanoma type.

adjuvant therapy. A treatment offered in addition to the surgical removal of melanoma. Generally, the therapy is designed to affect the whole body and kill any disease that may have traveled to other parts of the body even before the primary tumor or diseased lymph nodes are recognized and removed.

anti-CTLA-4. A classification of therapies including IPI (ipi-limumab) and Yervoy that act to put the brakes on tumor growth by becoming immune boosters. They block a protein called CTLA-4 that acts as a brake on T cells, the soldiers of the immune system. These therapies were approved by the FDA in March 2011 for use in stage IV patients.

anti-PD-1. A promising immunotherapy approved by the FDA in September 2014 for use in stage IV melanoma.

basal cell carcinoma (BCC). One of the two most common kinds of nonmelanoma cancer. It almost never metastasizes and is made up of the cells at the bottom layer of the epidermis that give rise to keratinocytes.

biopsy. Surgical removal of a sample of tissue for examination under a microscope.

B-raf. The B-raf protein is a key component of the cellular pathways and may become mutated and cause tumor growth. New *BRAF* therapies target this mutation to eliminate tumor progression.

carcinogen. A chemical, physical, or biological agent that causes cancer.

CAT, or CT, Scan. Computerized tomography, An X-ray procedure in which a computer produces detailed pictures of areas inside the body.

chemotherapy. A form of therapy that uses medicines prescribed by medical oncologists to kill cancer cells directly. Given by pill or intravenously. It is a systemic therapy since it travels through the bloodstream to reach the entire body.

congenital nevi. Moles that are present at birth; sometimes called birthmarks.

dermatopathologist. A physician who has special training in diagnosing disease on the basis of microscopic examination of the skin.

dermis. The layer of skin directly beneath the epidermis.

dysplastic nevi (DN). Moles associated with an increased risk of melanoma. Larger than ordinary moles, they are flat or have a flat part, have indistinct or fuzzy borders, and are often uneven in coloration.

epidermis. The outermost layer of skin.

excisional biopsy. A biopsy in which all of a tumor in evidence is taken off.

FDA (Food andDrug Administration). The federal government agency responsible for approval of the use of certain drugs used as therapies.

immunotherapy. A treatment designed to help your body's immune system fight cancer, similar to how your body fights off infections.

incisional biopsy. A biopsy done with a knife, sampling only a part of a lesion.

interferon (INF). A type of protein produced naturally by the immune system. Also refers to a group of synthetic treatments, including one for stage III melanoma called Intron A, which is FDA approved.

interleukin-2. A type of protein molecule produced by lymphocytes that activates other lymphocytes in the immune system. Approved by the FDA, the artificially made treatment is called IL-2, or Proleukin, and is sometimes prescribed for stage IV disease.

lesion. A well-defined, localized abnormality within an organ—for example, a pigmented growth on the skin.

lymph gland/lymph node. Small, bean-shaped organs located in the lymphatic system.

lymphocyte. A type of white blood cell that plays an important part in immune reactions.

lymphoscintigraphy. A technique in which a small amount of radioactive material is injected near the site of a primary melanoma then different lymph node areas (armpits and groin, for example) are scanned to see which group(s) of nodes "light up."

magnetic resonance imaging (MRI). An imaging study that uses a magnetic field and a computer to create detailed pictures of the body.

melanocytes. Cells located primarily at the bottom of the epidermis that transfer pigment to other cells. Responsible in part for skin and hair color.

MEK inhibitor. A chemical or drug that inhibits the mitogen-activated protein kinase enzymes MEK1 and/or MEK2. The inhibitor can be used to affect the MAPK/ERK pathway, which is often overactive in some cancers. MEK inhibitors have potential to treat some cancers, especially *BRAF*-mutated melanoma, and are being tried on *BRAF*-negative patients, too.

metastases. Spread of cancer cells from one part of the body to another.

National Cancer Institute (NCI). Federally funded cancer research and treatment center run by the National Institutes of Health (NIH).

nevus (plural is nevi). A mole.

no evidence of disease (NED). Classification indicating that there is no measurable evidence of melanoma in your body.

palliative care. Treatment that is intended to relieve symptoms but not cure disease.

pathology. The science of diagnosing disease by such methods as microscopic analysis of tissue.

PET scan (positron emission tomography). A radioactive tracer attached to a sugar that is injected into the patient to find areas of tumor activity.

pigmented lesion. A skin spot that has color—brown, black, or blue.

primary tumor or site. Initial tumor or the site on the body where it forms.

punch biopsy. A biopsy in which a cookie-cutter-like instrument is used to cut out a core of tissue.

radial growth phase (RGP). The earliest step in the development of melanoma, in which the disease is confined to the epidermis or barely penetrates the dermis. No cluster of melanoma cells forms and no metastases result.

regional perfusion therapy. A therapy in which an entire limb is infused with cancer-killing drugs. The drugs are introduced into the artery supplying the limb and are taken out through the vein. The technique may be used for melanoma when there are multiple skin metastases that are apparently confined to the arm or leg that was the site of the primary tumor.

seborrheic keratosis. A benign skin lesion associated with aging and sun exposure; not precancerous.

sentinel-node biopsy (SNB or SLNB). A type of biopsy in which a small amount of radioactive dye is injected into the area of the primary melanoma to scan for melanoma cells in the sentinel nodes.

shave biopsy. A biopsy done by shaving off a piece of skin with a sterile razor blade.

squamous cell cancer (SCC). One of the two common kinds of nonmelanoma skin cancer, it is a malignancy that seldom metastasizes and is made up of keratinocytes in the epidermis.

stage (of cancer). A measure of the extent of a malignancy, arrived at by examining features of the primary tumor and searching for evidence of metastasis.

subcutis/subcutaneous tissue. A layer of fat located under the dermis.

targeted therapies. Newer therapies whose approach is based on knowing how cancer cells function. These therapies work to stop cancer cells from growing and/or to make other therapies work better. Some work by preventing the growth of new blood vessels needed to nourish the cancer. Others work to block the action of molecules on the surface of cancer cells.

tumorigenic. Having the capacity to produce spherical collections of cancer cells.

UV-A and UV-B rays. Different wavelengths of ultraviolet light. Both types are implicated in skin cancer, skin aging, and sunburn.

Vemurafenib. Commercial name for the *BRAF* therapy PLX4032 (see **Zelboraf**).

vertical growth phase. A step in the development of melanoma in which the disease shows evidence of growth as a lump in the dermis (see **tumorigenic**). This phase of melanoma may metastasize.

Yervoy. A type of immunotherapy, it is the commercial name for ipilimumbab (IPI) or anti-CTLA 4 (see **anti-CTLA 4**).

wide local excision (WLE). A reexcision of the primary site after the biopsy results have been interpreted.

Zelboraf. The commercial name for the *BRAF* therapy Vemurafenib.

About the Author

Catherine Poole experienced melanoma twenty-six years ago during her pregnancy. The lack of scientifically sound information for patients at that time drove her to collaborate on two melanoma books with her oncologist, Dr. DuPont Guerry, who headed the melanoma program at the University of Pennsylvania. The books brought Ms. Poole many patients seeking advice, and in 2002 she started the Melanoma International Foundation. The foundation has never steered away from its mission of directly empowering patients with knowledge so they can live the longest, highest-quality lives possible. Ms. Poole previously wrote about her experience choosing a nurse-midwife; she has been a healthy home writer for Rodale Press and a freelance writer for many magazines. In her free time, she loves operating her small farm and trail riding.

NOTES

Chapter 1 What Is Melanoma?

1   Wallace Clark, "The Skin," in John Farber and Emanuel Rubin, eds., *Pathology* (Philadelphia: Lippincott, 1988).

2   Ibid.

3   Karen Shideler, "This Type of Melanoma Killed Bob Marley," and "When Ultraviolet Rays of Sunshine Become Ultraviolent: Skin Cancers," *Philadelphia Inquirer*, August 1, 1994.

4   DuPont Guerry et al., "Lessons from Tumor Progression: The Invasive Radial Growth Phase of Melanoma Is Common, Incapable of Metastasis and Indolent," *Journal of Investigative Dermatology* 100 (1992): 3425–55.

Chapter 2: Who Gets Melanoma and Why?

1   Marianne Berwick, "Patterns of Sun Exposure That Are Important in Melanoma," in *Challenges in Melanoma* (Hoboken, NJ: Blackwell Scientific Publishers, 2002), 3–15.

2 Richard Gallagher et al., "The Epidemiology of Acquired Melanocytic Nevi," *Dermatoepidemiology* 13 (1995), 3.

3 "Genetics of Skin Cancer," National Cancer Institute. http://www.cancer.gov/cancertopics/pdq/genetics/skin/HealthProfessional/page4

4 Rona McKie et al., "Lack of Effect of Pregnancy on Outcome of Melanoma," *Lancet* 337 (1991), 653–5.

5 Elizabeth Holly, Rosemary Cress, and David Ahn, "Cutaneous Melanoma in Women: Reproductive Factors and Oral Contraceptive Use," American Journal of Epidemiology: 141 (1995), 943–50.

Chapter 3: Finding Early Melanoma

1 American Cancer Society, "Cancer Facts & Figures 2014" American Cancer Society, (Atlanta, Georgia).

2 DuPont Guerry, Synnestvedt, Elder, and Schultz, "Lessons from Tumor Progression: The Invasive Radial Growth Phase Is Common, Incapable of Metastases, and Indolent," *Journal of Investigative Dermatology* 100, no. 3 (March 1993), 342S–345S.

3 Marianne Berwick et al., "Screening for Cutaneous Melanoma by Skin Self-Examination," *Journal of the National Cancer Institute* 88 (1996), 17–23.

Chapter 4: If You Have Melanoma

1 Lynn Schuchter et al., "A Prognostic Model for Predicting 10-Year Survival in Patients with Primary

Melanoma," *Annals of Internal Medicine* 125 (September 1996)1893-1904

2 DuPont Guerry, et., al A Population Based Validation of the AJCC Melanoma Staging System, 2004: ASCO Annual Meeting, Abstract 7500

3 Donald Morton, MD, et al, Final Trial Report of Sentinel Node Biopsy Versus Nodal Observation in Melanoma. New England Journal of Medicine 370: 599-609 February 13, 2104.

4 C.K Bichakjian, et al, "Melanoma Information on the Internet: Often Incomplete-A Public Health Opportunity," Journal of Clincial Oncology 20 (2002):1177

Chapter 5: When Melanoma Metastasizes

1 John Kirkwood et al., "Interferon Alfa-2b Adjuvant Therapy of High-Risk Resected Cutaneous Melanoma: The Eastern Cooperative Oncology Group Trial," *Journal of Clinical Oncology* 14 (1996), 7–17.

2 John Kirkwood et al., "Update on Adjuvant Interferon Therapy for High-Risk Melanoma," *Oncology* 16, no. 9, 1177. September,2002

3 Flaherty and Schuchter, "The Agarwala/Kirkwood Article Reviewed," *Oncology* 16, no. 9, 1177. September,2002.

4 Verma, Petrella, Hamm, Bak, and Charette, "Biochemotherapy for the Treatment of Metastatic Malignant Melanoma," *Current Oncology*, April 2008, 85–9, http://www.ncbi.nlm.nih.gov/pmc/articles/PMC2365480/.

[5] Keith Flaherty, MD, the director of the Henri and Belinda Termeer Center for Targeted Therapies at the Massachusetts General Hospital Cancer Center provided editorial oversight of this section.

[6] Jedd Wolchok, MD, the chief of the Melanoma and Immunotherapeutics Service at Memorial Sloan Kettering Cancer Center provided professional editorial oversight of this section.

[7] Kathleen M. Foley and Hellen Gelband, eds., *Improving Palliative Care for Cancer* (Washington, DC: National Academy Press, 2001).

Chapter 7: Tending to Your Spirits

[1] David Spiegel, "Effect of Psychosocial Treatment on Survival of Patients with Metastatic Breast Cancer," *Lancet* 14, no. 2 (October 1989), 888–90.

[2] Fawzy Fawzy, "Malignant Melanoma: Effects of an Early Structured Psychiatric Intervention, Coping, and Affective State on Recurrence and Survival, Six Years Later," *Archives of General Psychiatry* (Aug. 1990): 681–9.

[3] Pettigrew, Thomas, et al. Nov 9, 2002, British Medical Journal. http://www.bmj.com/content/vol325/issue 7372).

INDEX

ABCDEs of early detection, 7, 32

Abscesses, 58

Abscopal effect, 87

Acral lentiginous melanoma, 5, 11, 35, 104, 119

ACS. *See* American Cancer Society

ACT (adoptive cell transfer), 85–87, 109

Acupuncture, 91

ADC therapy (DEDN6526A), 111

Adjuvant therapy, 63, 72–77

Adoptive cell therapy (ACT), 85–87, 109

Age

    and melanoma, 9

    and skin changes, 10, 13

Ahn, David, 23

AJCC. *See* American Joint Committee on Cancer

Alternative medicine, 91–92

Amelanotic melanoma, 6

American Cancer Society, 27, 33

American Joint Committee on Cancer (AJCC), 48, 50

American Medical Association (AMA) on tanning salons, 13

American Psychological Oncology Society (APOS), 117

Antianxiety medications, 127

Anti-CTLA-4 antibodies, 83–84. *See also* Ipilimumab (IPI; Yervoy)

Antidepressant medications, 127

Antigens, 82

Anxiety, 121, 122, 127

Artificial tanning, 13–14

Asymmetry in moles 7, 32

Atypical moles (dysplastic nevi), 16–17, 19

Australia

    melanoma rates in 24, 53

    melanoma treatment in, 83

Axillary nodes, 54

Basal cell carcinoma, 4, 9, 25, 43

Berwick, Marianne 30

Biochemotherapy, 76

Biological therapies, 77–78

Biopsies

    deep shave, 42

    determining need for, 44

    excisional, 42, 44

    incisional, 43

    initial, 59, 98–99

    needle, 105

    punch, 42–43

results of, 115–116

sentinel lymph node, 51–2, 53–57, 108, 111, 112

See also Pathology reports

Birth control pills, 23–24

Birthmarks. *See* Congenital nevi

Bleeding, 35

Blood blisters, 4

Blood vessels, 3

Bloodwork, 58

Body, worrying about, 125–126

Border irregularity in moles 7, 32

Bottled tans, 14

BRAF gene mutation, 12, 63, 72

BRAF inhibitor-based therapy, 77, 78–82, 85, 86, 105–106

B-raf protein, 80–81, 105

Brain involvement

lesions, 112–113

metastases, 5, 71, 78, 88, 95, 111, 112

radiation treatment, 107–108, 111

tumors, 107

Breast cancer, 73, 120

Breastfeeding, 102

Breathing exercises, 126–127

Breslow, Alexander, 46

Breslow levels, 56, 61, 121

British Columbia Cancer Agency, 15

Bush, Barbara, 36

Bush, George H.W., 36–37

Cancer
    breast, 73, 120
    myths about, 43, 124
    prostate, 91
    psychological factors affecting 120, 121
    See also Melanoma; Skin cancer
Cancer Information Service hotline, 100
Carcinogens, 10, 28
Caregivers, emotional support for, 117
Caregiving, 93–96
CAT (computerized axial tomography) scans, 58, 70, 105, 107
Center for Mindfulness in Medicine, 119
Chemotherapy, 73, 76, 77–78, 86, 88
    negative interactions with, 91–92
Chest x-rays, 58, 62, 70
Chiang, Veronica, 108
Children
    and germline mutation, 19
    with melanoma, 20
    moles on, 15, 16
    and sun exposure, 12
C-kit mutation, 82
Clark, Wallace, 2, 6, 99, 100–101
Clarks' Level, 47
Clinical trials
    for adjuvant therapies, 76, 77, 78, 85, 87, 109, 110, 111
    concurrent with hospice care, 93
    double-blind, 90

exclusions from, 107

finding, 63, 68, 77, 88–89, 110, 118

phases of, 89

questions to ask, 89–91

randomized, 89–90

Cobas HPV test, 80

Color variation in moles, 7, 32

Complete node dissection, 55

Comprehensive Cancer Centers, 69

Congenital nevi (moles), 16

Connor, Stephen, 112–113

Coping styles, 124–125

mind-body therapies, 91, 124–25

Costs

of screening, 28, 38

of treatment, 75, 84, 86

Counseling, 94, 117, 124

Cress, Rosemary, 23

CT (computed tomography) scans, 58, 70, 105, 107

CTLA-4, 83

Cure *See* Treatment

CyberKnife, 108

Cytokines, 78

Dabrafenib, 80

Dacarbazine (DTIC), 77–78, 89, 107, 109

Death, 58, 93, 95–96, 116

Death rates from melanoma, 27, 121

DEDN6526A, 111

Deep shave biopsy, 42

Denial, 35, 118, 124

Depression, 121, 127

Dermatologists, 34, 42, 59, 98

Dermatopathologists, 45, 46

Dermis, 2, 3, 7, 29

Diagnosis, delay in, 35

Diagnostic tests, 58

Diameter greater than 6mm, 7, 32

Dihydroxyacetone (DHA), 14

Dissections. *See* Lymph nodes; Sentinel lymph nodes

Disseminated melanoma, 77

Distant metastases, 71

Doctors. *See* Dermatologists; dermatopathologists; Health care professionals; Oncologists; Pathologists; Plastic surgeons; Psychologists

Drug comparisons, ineffective, 89

Drug therapy, 28, 78. *See also* Adjuvant therapies; Clinical trials

DTIC (dacarbazine), 77–78, 89, 107, 109

Dye, injection of, 54

Dysplastic nevi (atypical moles), 9, 16–17, 19, 29, 31, 34
    Nonmelanoma, 46

Early detection
    ABCDEs, 7, 32
    current statistics, 27–28

finding early melanoma, 29–30

free screening programs, 38

location, 34–35

professional examination, 30, 33–34

skin examination, 30–33

targeting those at risk, 39

warning others, 35–38

Elderly, lentigo maligna melanoma in, 5

Elective lymph node dissection, 52–53

Elevation of melanoma, 7, 32. See also Thickness of melanoma

England, melanoma rates in, 21

Epidermis, 3, 4, 7, 14, 29, 47

Europe, 24, 83

Examination of skin. *See* Self-examination, skin

"Examine Your Skin," 31

Excision, size of, 57–58

Excisional biopsy, 42, 44

Exercise, 91

Extremities

melanoma located on, 21

swelling of, 52

Eyes, melanoma in 6

Family, 121, 123–124

Family history, 9, 29, 34, 39

Fawzy, F.I., 121

Flaherty, Keith, 86

Flat (radial growth) stage. *See* Radial growth (nontumorigenic) phase
Follow-up, 16, 30, 51, 59, 61, 90, 102, 107, 118
Food and Drug Administration (FDA) approval
    of adjuvant therapies, 76
    of *BRAF* and MEK inhibitors 80, 81
    of DTIC, 78
    of immunologic agents, 83
    of interferon, 74
    of IPI, 83
    of Keytruda, 85
Freckles, 11, 39
Friedlaender, Jonathan, 111–112
Friends, 121, 123–124

Gallagher, Richard, 15
Gamma Knife, 108, 112
Garment nevi (moles), 16
Gender-based predisposition, 9, 21
Genes
    BRAF, 12, 63, 72
    mutant, 19–20, 79, 80–82
    RAF kinase, 79
Geography, as predisposing factor, 9, 24–25
Germline mutation, 19
Giant congenital nevi, 16
Glossary of terms, 129–35
Goldfarb, Jamie Troil, 108–109

Granulocyte macrophage colony-stimulating factor
(GM-CSF; Leukine; Sargramostim), 76, 107–108
Grieving, 95, 96, 125
Growth phase. *See* Radial growth (nontumorigenic) phase;
Vertical (tumorigenic) phase
Guerry, DuPont, 28, 50, 64, 100, 102–104, 126
on curable melanoma, 28
on lymph node examination, 64
on survival rates 50
treatment of Catherine Poole, 100, 102–4, 126
Guilt, 118, 124–25

Hair associated with mole, 16
Hair color, 11, 20
Handley, William, 57
Health care issues, 37–38, 41–42, 75–76
Health care professionals
finding a doctor, 59, 68–69
identification of lesions by, 41–42
questions regarding lymph node involvement, 56–57
questions regarding suspicious skin growth, 43–44
screening for melanoma by, 37–39
See also Dermatologists; Dermatopathologists; Oncologists;
Pathologists; Plastic surgeons; Psychologists
Health insurance, 75, 86, 90, 93, 94, 117
Health on the Net (HON) Foundation, 66
Heredity. *See* Family history
Holly, Elizabeth, 23

Hormonal therapy, 73

Hormone replacement therapy (HRT), 23–24

Hormones

immunological, 78

skin changes due to, 34

Hospice care, 92–94

Houlden, Arlene, 117–118, 125

Hypervigilance, 125

IL-2 (interleukin-2), 76, 78, 82, 86, 105, 110, 111, 112

Immune system, 82–83, 86, 121, 126

Immunological hormones, 78

Immunotherapies, 28, 72, 77, 82–85, 86, 87

Improving Palliative Care for Cancer, 94

In situ melanoma, 7, 29, 59

Incisional biopsy, 43

Ineffective drug comparisons, 89

Inflammation, 58

Infrared radiation, 10

Inguinal nodes, 54

Interferon alfa-2b (Intron A), 63, 74–76, 82, 107, 111

Interleukin-2 (IL-2), 76, 78, 82, 86, 105, 110, 111, 112

Internal organ involvement, 49, 58, 77

Internet information, 12, 65–68, 123

Intralesional therapies, 72

Intron A (interferon alfa-2b), 63, 74–76, 82, 107, 111

Ipilimumab (IPI; Yervoy), 77, 83–84, 87, 110, 111, 112

Itching of melanomas, 34

Kabat-Zinn, Jon, 119

Kaminski, Richard, 105–106

Keratinocytes, 3, 4

Keratosis, seborrheic, 44, 46

Keytruda, 84–85, 111. *See also* PD-1 immunotherapies

Kinase inhibitors. *See BRAF* therapies; Molecularly targeted therapy

Laser surgery, 71

Lentigo maligna melanoma, 5, 13

Lesions

    brain, 112–13

    low-risk, 61

    lung, 113

    melanoma, 18, 52, 56, 59, 60, 72, 112

    primary, 61

    See also Melanoma styles

Leukine (GM-CSF; Sargramostim), 76, 107–8

Level of invasion (Clark's level), 47

Lumpy (vertical growth) phase. *See* Vertical growth (tumorigenic) phase

Lymph, 50

Lymph nodes

    axillary, 54

    complete node dissection, 55

    defined, 50

    dissection of, 52–53, 57, 73, 111

    elective dissection of, 52–53

inguinal, 54

involvement of, 47–52, 56–57, 58, 61, 62, 63, 70, 73, 107

mapping of, 54–57

self-exams, 64

swollen/enlarged, 52–53, 57

See also Sentinel lymph nodes

Lymph vessels, 3, 50, 67

Lymphedema, 105

Lymphocytes, 51. *See also* Tumor-infiltrating lymphocytes

Lymphoscintigraphy, 54

Malignancy, 3, 10, 79. *See also* Cancer; Melanoma

Managed care, 37

Mandela, Nelson, 115

Margin, 60

Marley, Bob, 5

MD Anderson Cancer Center, 87

Medical oncologists. *See* Oncologists

Medical photographers, 59

Medical records, 45

Meditation, 91, 126

mindful, 119

MEK inhibitors, 80–82

Mekinist, 80

Melanin pigment, 3, 10, 20

absence of, 6

Melanocytes, 3, 15, 20, 28

abnormal, 7

Melanoma

    appearance of, 4–5, 7, 32, 34

    in the dermis, 3

    disseminated, 77

    elevation of, 7, 32

    family history of, 9, 29, 34, 39

    gender-based predisposition toward, 9, 21

    hereditary aspects of, 19–21

    and hormones, 23

    in situ, 7, 29, 59

    location of, 34–35, 47

    and moles, 17–18

    origin of, 3

    and pregnancy, 22, 97, 98–104

    prognosis of, 46–48

    psychological stress of, 115–117

    radial growth (nontumorigenic) phase, 6–7, 18, 28, 46–47, 52, 59, 61

    skin types susceptible to, 9–11

    stages of, 48–50

    survival rate for, 48–50, 53, 63, 74, 100–101

    thickness of, 47, 48, 53, 56

    vertical growth (tumorigenic) phase, 7, 28–29, 46–47, 60, 61–62

    when it is curable, 28–29

    See also Early detection; Risk factors; Treatment

Melanoma diagnosis

    biopsies, 42–43

pathology reports, 44–45

second opinions, 45

Melanoma International Foundation (MIF), 88, 100, 104

MIF website, 31, 66, 67, 69, 98, 108, 123

Melanoma locations

arms, 21

backs, 4, 30, 31, 34, 54

breasts, 17

buttocks, 17

extremities, 21

feet, 5, 31

fingernails, 5, 31

hands, 5, 31

head, 21

legs, 21

on men, 4, 13, 17, 34

toenails, 5, 31

trunk, 21

on women, 4, 17, 34

Melanoma stages

for support groups, 123

stage I, 48, 58, 97

stage II, 48, 73, 97, 98–104

stage III, 49, 63, 76, 77, 97, 104–105

stage IV, 49, 76, 77, 78, 105–106, 109–110, 111–112

stage V, 49

Melanoma types

acral lentiginous melanoma, 5, 11, 35, 104, 119

amelanotic melanoma, 6

lentigo maligna melanoma, 5, 13

metastatic, 28–29, 85

mucosal melanoma, 5, 11, 35

nodular melanoma, 4, 12, 18

ocular melanoma, 6

superficial spreading, 4, 12, 23, 35

Men

incidence of melanoma in, 21, 27

life expectancy of, 99, 120

location of melanomas on, 4, 13, 17, 34

Menopausal hormone replacement 23–24

Mental health professionals, 68

psychologists, 59

therapists, 117, 127

Metastasis

adjuvant therapies, 72–73

defined, 69–70

distant, 71

likelihood of, 52

in the lungs, 107

in the lymph nodes, 56, 61

regional, 70–71

in the skin, 61

types of, 70–71

use in determining stage of melanoma, 48

See also Brain involvement

Mind-body connection, 124–125

Mind-body therapies, 91

Mindfulness, 119

Mitotic count, 48

Moffitt Cancer Center, 87

Mohs, Frederick E., 43

Mohs micrographic surgery, 43

Molecularly targeted therapies, 78–82. *See also BRAF* therapies

Moles (nevi), 4, 15–18

    atypical, 16–17, 19

    changes in, 16, 18–19, 32–33, 93

    congenital, 16

    dysplastic, 9, 16–17, 19, 29, 31, 34, 46

    garment nevi, 16

    giant congenital nevi, 16

    ordinary/normal/common (benign), 9, 31, 34, 44, 46, 81

    as precursors to melanoma, 4, 17

    removal of, 18–19

    as risk factor, 15, 17

Mortality rates, 21, 121

Morton, Donald, 56

MRI (magnetic resonance imaging), 58

Mucosal melanoma, 5, 11, 35

Myths about cancer, 43, 124

National Cancer Institute (NCI)

    Cancer Information Service hotline, 100

    clinical trials, 77, 85, 88

    designation of Comprehensive Cancer Centers by, 69

Journal of, 30

studies of heredity, 19–20

TIL therapy at, 86

and treatment with interleukin-2, 78

National Institutes of Health (NIH), 86, 109

NCI. *See* National Cancer Institute

Neurotropism, 60

Never Walk This Path Alone (video), 98, 113

Nevi. *See* Moles

Nivolumab (Opdivo), 85

Nodular melanoma, 4, 12, 18

Nontumorigenic (radial growth) phase. *See* Radial growth (nontumorigenic) phase

Nonwhites, melanoma in, 5, 10–11

NRAS mutation, 81

Nursing care, 94

Nursing staff, 69

Ocular melanoma, 6

Oncogenes, 12

Oncologists, 59, 68, 73, 88, 90, 108

    questions for, 63–64

    surgical, 59, 90

Oncology, psychological, 117–118

Oncology Drug Advisory Council, 74

Opdivo (Nivolumab), 85

Oral contraceptives, 23–24

Pain management, 57, 61, 101–102

Palliative care, 64, 92–96

Papillary dermis, 3

Pathologists, 44–45, 46, 68

Pathology reports, 44–45, 57, 99

    questions about, 46

    slides, 45

Patient experiences

    Stephen Connor, 112–113

    Jonathan Friedlaender, 111–112

    Jamie Troil Goldfarb, 108–109

    Richard Kaminski, 105–106

    Catherine Poole, 98–104

    T.J. Sharpe, 109–110

    Alicia Tagliaferro, 106–108

    Shirley Zaremba, 104–105

Patients

    effect of age on prognosis, 47, 77

    effect of sex on prognosis, 47

    emotional support for, 117

    high-risk, 45, 61–62, 73

    histories of, 47, 77, 103

    involvement of, 116–117

    low-risk, 61

    See also Patient experiences

PD-1 immunotherapies, 77, 84–85, 87, 110, 111, 112

Persons of color, 5, 10–11

PET (positron emission tomography) scans, 58, 70, 105

Pettigrew, M., 125

Pharmaceuticals, 28, 78

Photography for screening, 19, 34, 103

Physicians. *See* Dermatologists; Dermatopathologists; Health care professionals; Oncologists; Pathologists; Plastic surgeons; Psychologists

Pig skin, 2–3

Pigmented Lesion Clinic (Pigmented Lesion Group), 19, 35, 47, 61, 102

Placebos, 89, 90

Plastic surgeons, 43, 59

Post-traumatic stress disorder (PTSD), 94

Pregnancy, 22, 97, 98–104

Prophylactic lymph node dissection, 52–53

Prostate cancer, 91

Psychological oncology, 117–118

Psychological services, 117

Psychological support, effect on cancer, 120, 121

Psychologists, 59. *See also* Mental health professionals

Punch biopsy, 42–43

PV-10, 72

Quality of life, 121–122

Questions to ask

about clinical trials, 89–91

for health care professionals, 43–44

for the oncologist, 63–64

about pathology report, 46

about regional lymph node involvement, 56–57

for the surgeon, 60–61

Radial growth (nontumorigenic) phase, 6–7, 18, 28, 46–47, 52, 59, 61

diagnosis of, 46–47

in situ, 6

invasive, 6

and lymph node dissection, 52

melanomas that skip, 18

risk factor for, 61

treatment of, 28, 59

Radiation

infrared, 10

ultraviolet, 3, 10, 11–12, 13

visible, 10

Radiation therapy, 63, 72–73, 87

negative interactions with 91–92

stereotactic, 111

Radioactive solution, injection of, 54, 58

RAF kinase genes, 79

Randomized trials, 89–90. *See also* Clinical trials

Recurrence, 105, 108, 115, 126

chance of, 64

Regional metastases, 70–71

Regional perfusion therapy, 71

Relaxation techniques, 91, 127

Remissions, 77, 78, 85

Reticular dermis, 3
Risk factors
    age, 9
    family history of skin cancer or melanoma, 9, 19–21, 39
    gender, 9, 21
    geography, 9, 24
    having "funny-looking" moles, 9, 16–17, 39
    having many moles, 9, 15–18, 39
    history of skin cancer or melanoma, 9, 39
    history of sun overexposure, 9, 11–13, 21
    oral contraceptive use, 23–24
    pregnancy, 22
    skin type, sun-sensitive, 9, 11, 21, 39
    use of tanning salons, 13–14
Rosenberg, Stephen, 78

Sargramostim (Leukine; GM-CSF), 76, 107–8
Schuchter, Lynn, 47
Scotland, melanoma rates in, 21
Screening programs, 38–39
Seborrheic keratosis, 44, 46
Second opinions, 45, 68
Self-esteem, 122
Self-examinations
    lymph node, 64
    skin, 29–33, 39
Sentinel lymph nodes
    biopsies, 51–57, 108, 111, 112

pros and cons of biopsies, 55–57

sampling of, 54–57

See also Lymph nodes

Sharpe, T.J., 109–110

Shave biopsies, 42

Side effects

of clinical trial treatments, 90

of interferon, 74–75

of IPI (Yervoy), 83–84

of MEK inhibitors, 82

of PD-1 (Keytruda), 84–85

Skin

aging effect of sunlight on, 10, 13, 15

changes in 32–34

effects of aging on, 10

protective role of, 2

social role of, 2

structure of, 3

sun-damaged, 12–13

of swine, 2–3

types of, 11, 20, 39

Skin cancer

basal cell, 4, 9, 20, 25, 43

family history of, 9, 29, 34, 39

gender-based predisposition to, 9, 21

geography as predisposing factor, 9, 24–25

nonmelanoma, 13, 15

squamous cell, 4, 9, 20, 25, 43

See also Melanoma

Skin examinations
    free screenings, 38
    professional, 30, 33–34, 39, 41–42
    self-, 29–33, 39
Skin grafts, 60, 101
Soy supplements, 91
Spiegel, David, 120–121
Spray-on tans, 14
Squamous cell carcinoma, 4, 9, 20, 25, 43
St. John's wort, 91
Staging System (AJCC), 48–49, 50
Stereotactic radiation (SRS), 111
Stinging of melanomas, 34
Stress Reduction Clinic, 119
Subcutis, 3
Sun exposure
    aging effects of, 15
    beneficial, 14–15
    as cause of melanoma, 4, 5, 11–13
    childhood, 12, 20, 24–25
    cultural shift in attitude toward, 1, 12–15
    protection from 33
    See also Sun tanning; Sunburns
Sun lamps, 25
Sun sensitivity, 4, 9
Sun tanning, 1, 9, 10
Sunburns, 4, 10, 11

childhood, 15, 103

Superficial spreading melanoma, 4, 12, 23, 35

Support groups, 91, 106, 120–123

    locations for, 122–123

    web-based, 123

Surgeons, 59, 68, 99, 101, 108

    questions for, 60–61

Surgery

    inpatient, 57, 61

    laser, 71

    outpatient, 57, 61

    recovery from, 57

    size of excision, 57–58

    size of surgical wound, 59–60

Surgical oncologists, 59, 90. *See also* Oncologists

Survival rate, 48–50, 53, 63, 74, 100–101

Sylatron, 111

Tagliaferro, Alicia, 106–108

Talimogene laherparepvec (T-VEC), 72

Tanning, 1, 9, 10

    artificial, 13–14

Tanning salons, 13–14

T-cells, 82, 86

Temcad, 78

Temodal, 78

Temodar, 78

Temozolomide, 78

Therapeutic lymph node dissection. *See* Lymph nodes, dissection of

Therapists, 117, 127. *See also* Mental health professionals

Thickness of melanoma, 47, 48, 53, 56. *See also* Elevation of melanoma

TIL therapy, 85–87, 109, 110

Treatment

    abscopal effect, 87

    adjuvant therapies, 63, 72–77

    advanced stage, 28

    alternative medicine, 91–92

    BRAF therapies, 77, 78–82, 85, 86, 105–106

    chemotherapy and biological therapies, 73, 76, 77–78, 86, 88, 91–92

    cost of, 75, 84, 86

    for disseminated melanoma, 78

    for distant metastasis, 87

    immunotherapies, 28, 72, 77, 82–85, 86, 87

    intralesional therapies, 72

    lymph node dissection, 52–53, 55, 57, 73, 111

    more information, 65–66

    palliative care, 64, 92–96

    referral to an oncologist, 62–64

    for regional metastases, 71–72

    sentinel lymph node biopsies, 53–57, 108, 111, 112

    surgery, 57–61

    after surgery, 61–62

    TIL therapy, 85–87, 109, 110

See also Clinical trials

Tumorigenic (vertical growth) phase. *See* Vertical growth (tumorigenic) phase

Tumor-infiltrating lymphocytes (TILs), 85, 109

Tumors, 58

    BRAF gene mutation, 12, 63, 79, 80–81

    evaluation of, 48

    factors affecting, 47

    PET scans of, 58

    primary, 69–70, 72

    progression of, 17, 29, 44–49, 53

    treatment of, 62, 67, 73, 77, 82, 82, 83, 85, 86, 106, 109–110

    See also Vertical growth (tumorigenic) phase

Ulceration, 35

Ultraviolet radiation, 10, 11–12, 13

    wavelengths of, 3, 10

University of Pennsylvania, 19

UV-A and UV-B rays, 10, 11, 13

UV-C rays, 10

Vaccines, 78, 88

Vertical growth (tumorigenic) phase

    features of, 7

    prognosis of, 46–47

    progression of, 28–29

    risk factor for, 61

    surgery, 60

Visible radiation, 10
Vitamin A, 91
Vitamin C, 91
Vitamin D, 13, 14

Warts, changes in, 33
Whole-body photography, 19, 34, 103
Women
    and hormones, 23
    incidence of melanoma in, 21, 27
    location of melanomas on, 4, 17, 34
    and menopausal hormone replacement, 23–24
    and pregnancy, 22, 97, 98–104
    self-examination by, 30–31
    in support groups, 120
    survival rate of, 21, 99
World Health Organization (WHO), 13, 24
Worry, 35, 38, 45, 52, 84, 125–26

X-rays
    chest, 58, 62, 70
    diagnostic, 58

Yervoy (IPI; ipilimumab), 77, 83–84, 87, 110, 111, 112
Yoga, 91, 126

Zaremba, Shirley, 97, 104–105
Zelboraf, 80, 105–106